I0483124

biochemTEST

1000 multiple choice questions of biochemistry for university students

José Ramón Blas Pastor - PhD
(March' 2014)

Copyright © 2014 by JOSÉ RAMÓN BLAS PASTOR. All rights reserved.

Contact author at joseramonblas@gmail.com

Original title: "bqTEST: 1000 preguntas tipo test de bioquímica para universitarios"

First Edition: June 2013

First Edition of the English version: March 2014

Translated by: José Ramón Blas Pastor

ALL RIGHTS RESERVED. This book contains material protected under International Copyright Laws and Treaties. Any unauthorized reprint or use of this material is prohibited. No part of this publication may be reproduced, stored in a retrieval system, or transmitted in any form or by any means, electronic, mechanical, photocopying, recording, scanning, or by any information storage and retrieval system without express written permission from the author.

Index

Bioelements and main chemical groups

1. The four most abundant elements of living matter are...

- a. C, H, O, P
- b. C, O, S, P
- c. C, N, O, P
- d. C, O, H, N
- e. C, N, P, S

2. If we classify periodic table elements as follows...

- Group A. Those that must be ingested by humans, in normal conditions, in big quantities (some grams a day).
- Group B. Those that must be ingested by humans, in normal conditions, in small quantities (enough with some miligrams a day).
- Group C. those that are not needed by humans to maintain normal vital functions

... ¿which of the following lists does contain only elements of group A?

- a. C, N, O, F, P, S, Cl
- b. C, N, O, H, Be, Mg, Ca
- c. C, O, P, S, Cl, Na, K
- d. C, H, N, Fe, Cu, Zn, Mn
- e. C, N, P, S, Cu, Zn, Mg

3. Some chemical elements are essential for living beings, despite being present only at very small concentrations. For instance, an element called X, a metal, is found in the active site of hemocyanine, a protein involved in O_2 transport in many invertebrates. Which is this metal?

- a. iron
- b. nickel
- c. mercury
- d. copper
- e. zinc

4. Which of the following chemical groups is a thioester?

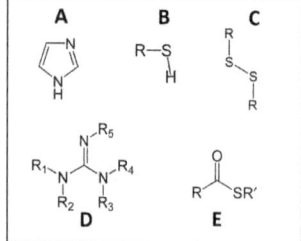

a. A
b. B
c. C
d. D
e. E

5. Which of the following values seems more reliable as a measure of the amount of iron in the organism of an adult alive person?

a. 2 ng
b. 2 µg
c. 2 mg
d. 2 g
e. 2 Kg

6. Some chemical elements are essential for living beings, despite being present only at very small concentrations. For instance, an element called X, a metal, is present in vitamin B_{12}. Which is this metal

a. iron
b. nickel
c. cobalt
d. palladium
e. platinum

7. Which of the following chemical groups is an imidazole?

A B C
D E

a. A
b. B
c. C
d. D
e. E

8. Which of the following chemical groups is a thiol?

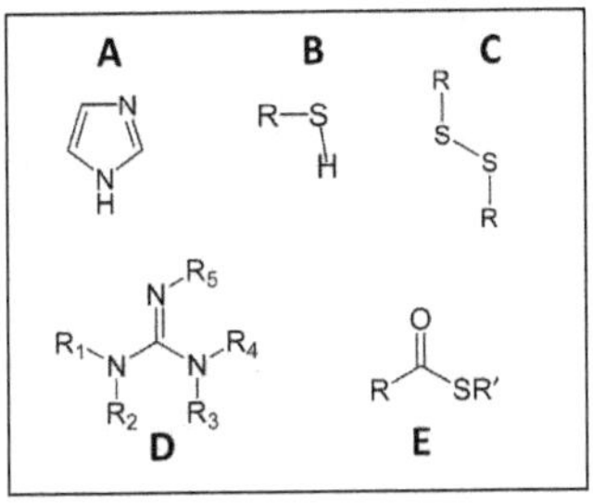

a. A
b. B
c. C
d. D
e. E

9. Almost all biological hydrogenases that oxidize molecular hydrogen (H_2) contain a metal in their active site, which is this metal?

a. lithium
b. cobalt
c. nickel
d. copper
e. platinum

10. Which of the following chemical groups is a disulfide?

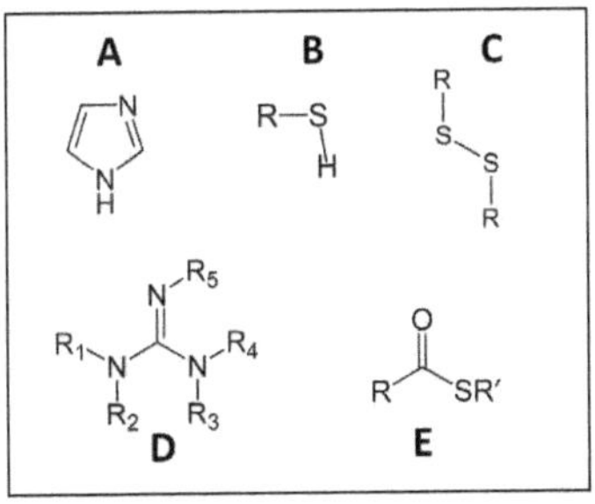

a. A
b. B
c. C
d. D
e. E

11. More than 65% of the iron present in human body is bound to a protein called...

a. cytochrome C
b. hemoglobin
c. actin
d. immunoglobulin
e. albumin

12. Which of the following chemical groups is an amine?

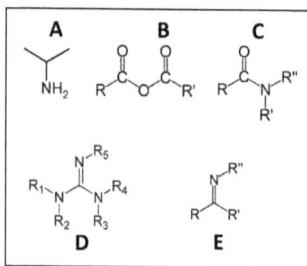

a. A
b. B
c. C
d. D
e. E

13. Urease is a bacterial enzyme that catalyzes conversion of urea into CO_2 and NH_3. When its structure was solved, in 1995, an important metal for catalysis was found at its active site. Which is this element?

a. nickel
b. palladium
c. lithium
d. lead
e. manganese

14. Which of the following chemical groups is an amide?

a. A
b. B
c. C
d. D
e. E

15. It has not been fully demonstrated that vanadium is an essential element for human beings. However, in the form of vanadate accompanying some drugs has proven to enhance the effects of a known hormone. Which is this hormone?

a. insulin
b. T4 (tetraiodothyronine)
c. adrenaline
d. testosterone
e. cortisol

16. Which of the following chemical groups is an imine?

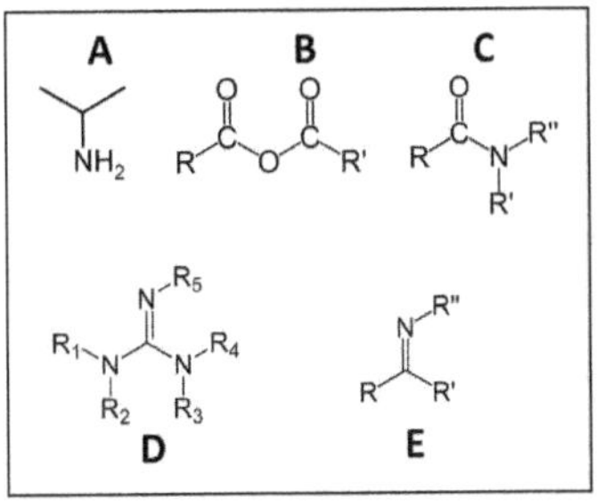

a. A
b. B
c. C
d. D
e. E

17. It has been discovered that some marine organisms accumulate vanadium in concentrations up to one million times higher than in surrounding water. This metal is accumulated by specific cells, mainly included in a molecule called hemovanadin. Which are these organisms?

a. sharks
b. lampreys
c. sea cucumbers
d. sea stars
e. tunicates

18. Boron is an essential element for many plants. Which of the following is its role?

a. It is a part of the active site in gibberellin receptor.
b. It strenghtens cell wall.
c. It has a role in transcription regulation of some genes.
d. It acts as a dielectric in mitochondrial membrane, allowing it to maintain a proton gradient during photosynthesis light-dependent reactions.
e. It acts in auxin signalling function, so being essential in shoot bud growth processes.

19. Which of the following chemical groups is an anhydride?

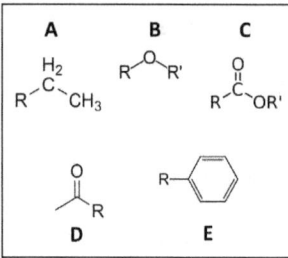

a. A
b. B
c. C
d. D
e. E

20. Which of the following foods has the highest amount of iron per unit of mass?

a. Full-cream milk
b. Yolk
c. Steak
d. Liver
e. Serrano ham

21. Which of the following chemical groups is an acetyl?

A   B   C

D   E

a. A
b. B
c. C
d. D
e. E

22. Some oxotransferases (enzymes dealing with oxidative processes) such as xanthine oxidase, aldehyde oxidase or nitrate reductase, contain the following cofactor at their active site.

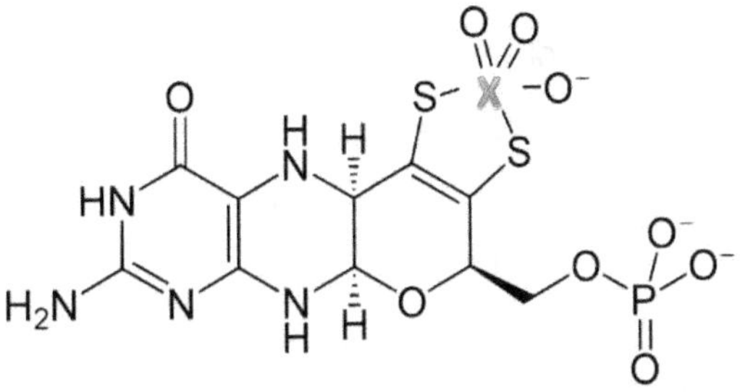

It is an heterocyclic compund that holds, in the X-labelled position, a metal scarcely found in living beings. Which is this element?

a. molybdenum
b. niobium
c. vanadium
d. nickel
e. lithium

23. Which of the following foods has the highest amount of iron per unit of mass?

a. Almonds
b. Hazlenuts
c. Walnuts
d. Pine nuts
e. Pistachios

24. An extremely important lowering of cupper concentration in human body is the cause of an strange hepatic pathology called...

a. Wilson's disease
b. Primary sclerosis cholangitis
c. Non-alcoholic fatty liver disease
d. Gilbert's syndrome
e. Crigler-Najjar syndrome

25. Which of the following chemical groups is a phenyl?

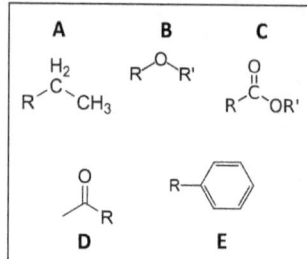

a. A
b. B
c. C
d. D
e. E

26. Some chemical elements are essential for living beings, although they are present only in very low concentrations. For instance, the element X, a methal, is present in the active site of haemoglobin, an O_2 transporting protein in vertebrates. Which is this methal?

a. iron
b. nickel
c. mercury
d. copper
e. zinc

27. Which of the following chemical group is an ester?

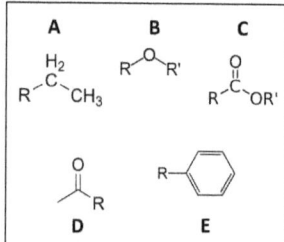

a. A
b. B
c. C
d. D
e. E

28. Which of the following chemical groups is an ether?

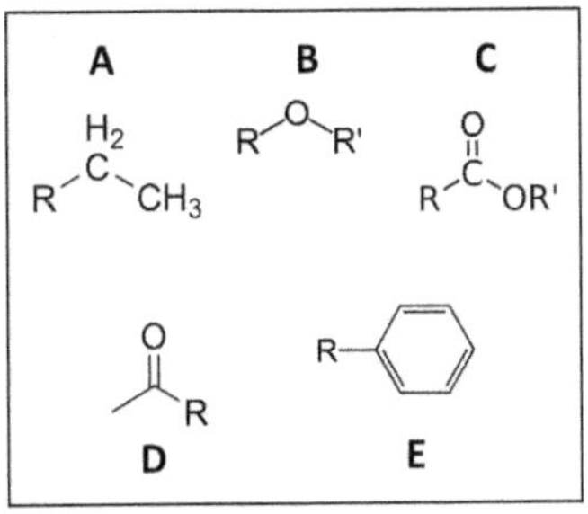

a. A
b. B
c. C
d. D
e. E

29. Which of the following chemical elements is an ethyl?

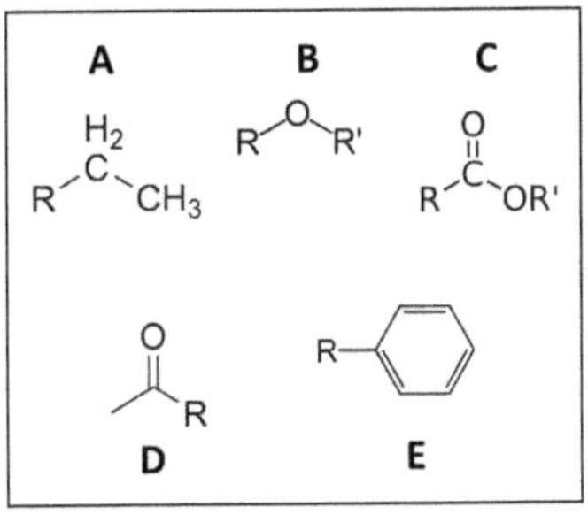

a. A
b. B
c. C
d. D
e. E

30. Ordered from highest to lowest abundancy, the five most abundant elements (when it comes to mass) of the Milky Way are...

a. hydrogen > helium > oxygen > carbon > neon
b. hydrogen > helium > oxygen > carbon > iron
c. hydrogen > oxygen > carbon > nitrogen > silicon
d. oxygen > hydrogen > carbon > nitrogen > silicon
e. hydrogen > oxygen > carbon > silicon > nitrogen

31. Ordered from highest to lowest abundancy, the two most abundant elements (when it comes to mass) of Earth's crust are...

a. hydrogen > oxygen
b. oxygen > silicon
c. hydrogen > aluminium
d. oxygen > nitrogen
e. hydrogen > carbon

32. Which of the following chemical groups is a methyl?

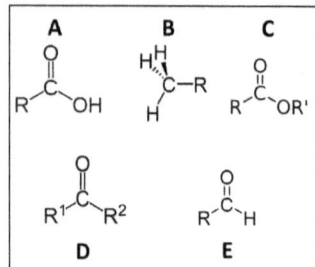

a. A
b. B
c. C
d. D
e. E

33. Which of the following chemical groups is an aldehyde?

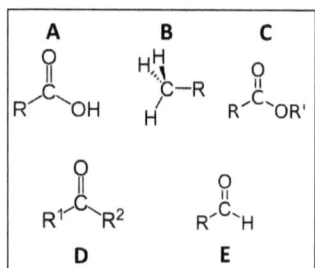

a. A
b. B
c. C
d. D
e. E

34. Which of the following chemical groups is a ketone?

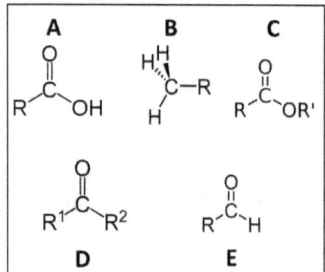

a. A
b. B
c. C
d. D
e. E

35. Which of the following lists does contain the chemical elements ordered from high to low according to their abundance (in mass) in the human body?

a. oxygen > hydrogen > nitrogen > sodium > calcium
b. oxygen > hydrogen > calcium > chlorine > cobalt
c. oxygen > carbon > phosphorus > potassium > fluorine
d. a and b are both right
e. b and c are both right

36. Which of the following chemical groups is a carboxyl?

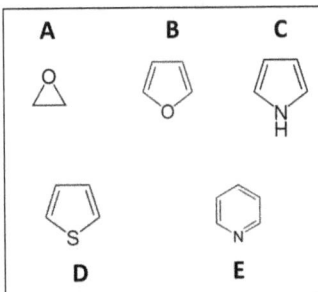

a. A
b. B
c. C
d. D
e. E

37. Which of the following molecules is a pyrrole?

a. A
b. B
c. C
d. D
e. E

38. Which of the following molecules is the furan?

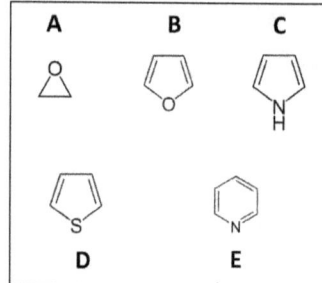

a. A
b. B
c. C
d. D
e. E

39. Which of the following molecules is the tiophene?

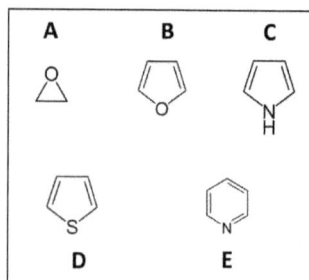

a. A
b. B
c. C
d. D
e. E

40. Which of the following molecules is a pyridine?

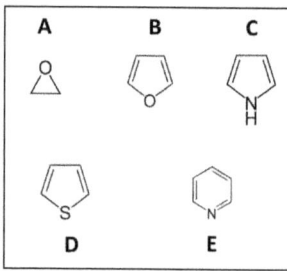

a. A
b. B
c. C
d. D
e. E

41. Which of the following molecules is an epoxide?

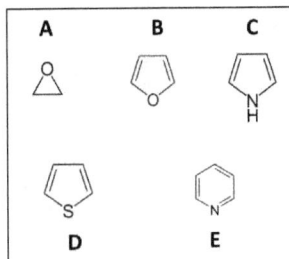

a. A
b. B
c. C
d. D
e. E

42. Which of the following molecules is the Acetyl-coenzyme A?

a. A
b. B
c. C
d. D
e. E

43. Which of the following molecules is the ATP?

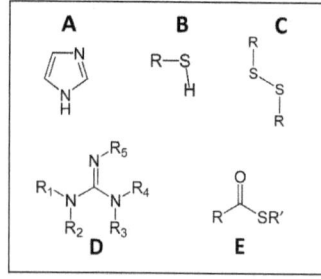

a. A
b. B
c. C
d. D
e. E

44. Which of the following chemical groups is a guanidinium?

a. A
b. B
c. C
d. D
e. E

45. Which of the following molecules is the phosphatidylcholine?

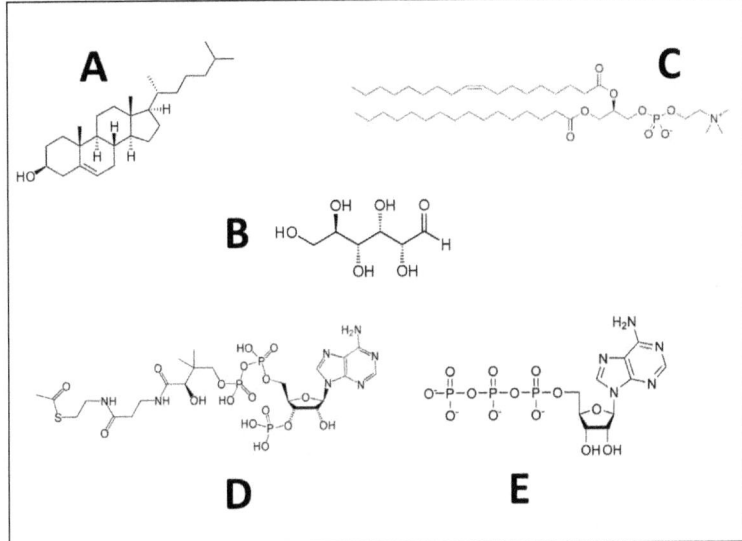

a. A
b. B
c. C
d. D
e. E

46. Among the following elements, which is the most abundant (in weight %) in human body?

a. calcium
b. phosphorous
c. sulphur
d. sodium
e. potassium

47. Which of the following molecules is the cholesterol?

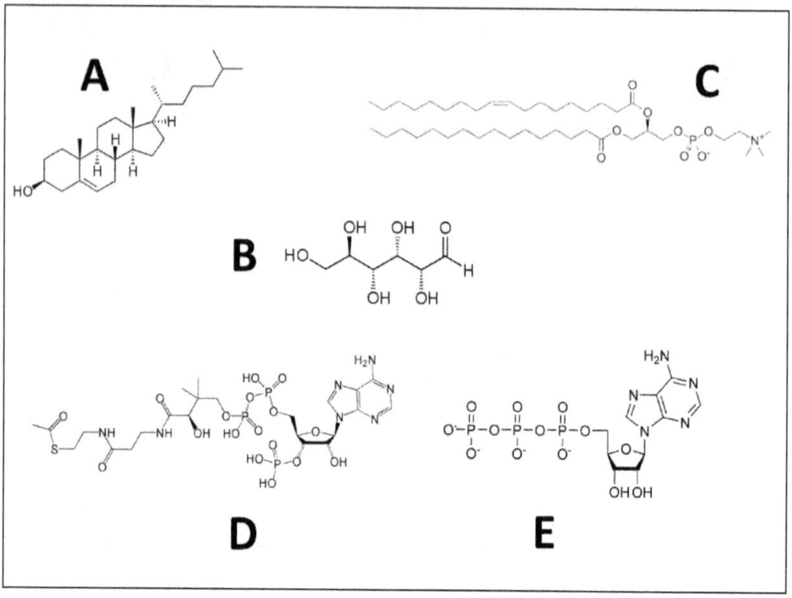

a. A
b. B
c. C
d. D
e. E

48. Among the following elements, which is the most abundant (in weight %) in human body?

a. copper
b. magnesium
c. sulphur
d. sodium
e. potassium

49. Which of the following molecules is glucose?

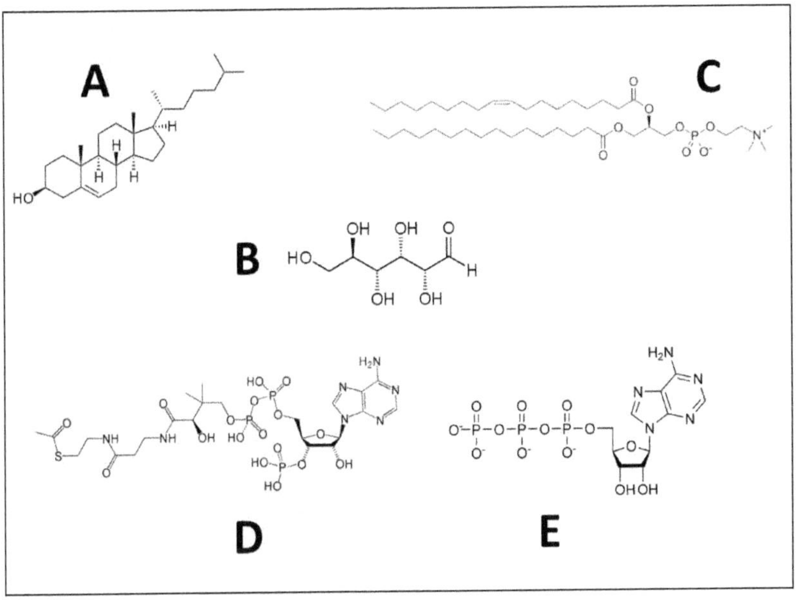

a. A
b. B
c. C
d. D
e. E

Water and mineral salts

50. Which is the average value for H-O-H angle of a water molecule at room temperature (25°C)?

    a. 104.5°
    b. 106.5°
    c. 109.5°
    d. 112.5°
    e. 120.5°

51. Water ...

    a. has an enthalpy of vaporization (heat energy needed to increase the temperature of 1 g of water by 1 °C) higher than other similar compounds such as H_2S or CH_4
    b. is denser in liquid state (at 3 °C) than in solid state
    c. has the melting point at a lower temperature than ammonia (NH_3)
    d. a, b and c are true
    e. a is false, b and c are true

52. Hydrogen bond produces an enthalpic stabilization of ...

    a. ~ 0.5 cal·mol^{-1}
    b. ~ 5 cal·mol^{-1}
    c. ~ 50 cal·mol^{-1}
    d. ~ 0.5 kcal·mol^{-1}
    e. ~ 5 kcal·mol^{-1}

53. If we compare water with an organic solvent, for instance, n-pentane, when it comes to viscosity (g/cm s) and surface tension (N/cm^2)...

    a. water presents a higher viscosity, but a lower surface tension
    b. water presents a lower viscosity and a lower surface tension
    c. water presents a higher viscosity and a higher surface tension
    d. water presents a lower viscosity, but a higher surface tension
    e. differences in viscosity and surface tension between both liquids are not significative (they are lower than a 10% of the higher value, in each case)

54. In the olden days, water was considered as a chemical element. It was in 1781 when it was discovered that it was a composed substance and not a single element. Who was the author of this discovery?

a. Antoine-Laurent de Lavoisier
b. James Watt
c. Isaac Newton
d. Claude Bernard
e. Henry Cavendish

55. In 1804, two scientists showed that water was composed by two volumes of hydrogen and one of oxygen. Who were them?

a. Antoine-Laurent de Lavoisier and Henry Cavendish
b. Joseph Louis Gauy-Lussac and Alexander von Humboldt
c. Isaac Newton and Robert Hooke
d. Henry Moseley and Dimtri Mendeleiev
e. Stephen Boltzmman and Jaques Dobbereiner

56. Water...

a. Is a polar molecule, where the highest negative charge density is located on oxygen
b. Is a polar molecule, where the highest negative charge density is located on hydrogens
c. Has a high dielectric constant if compared with apolar solvents such as hydrocarbons (n-pentane, n-hexane,...)
d. a and c are true
e. b and c are true

57. Indicate which sentence is FALSE. Water...

a. boils at a lower temperature on the top of Everest than at the sea level. Difference is around 30°C.
b. thanks to capilarity force, can advance in opposite direction than the one indicated by gravity force.
c. is a potent dielectric material, so its presence diminishes the 26ttractio of the force (electrostatic repulsion or 26ttraction) between two electric charges.
d. has a high surface tension, mainly due to its dipolar character and its ability to form hydrogen bonds.
e. as it has dissolved salts, it is a good conductor of electricity, an ability measured by a magnitude called conductivity. Sea water conductivity (measured in miliSiemens/m) is lower than the conductivity of drinking water.

58. Does the energy of interaction between a chloride anion and a sodium cation sepparated by 30 angstroms change if the chemical environment between them is water, ethanol or n-pentane, always at a temperature of 25°C? (Data: dielectric constant of water = 78,54 C^2/Nm^2, dielectric constant of ethanol = 24 C^2/Nm^2, dielectric constant of n-pentane = 1,84 C^2/Nm^2)

a. It does not vary considerably, since its value depends on temperature and not on the nature of the materials interposed between both charges.
b. It varies. The interaction is more intense in the case of water than in the case of n-pentane.
c. It would only vary if the temperature among solutions were also different.
d. It varies, being more intense as the apolar character of the solvent increases. In this case, intensity would decrese according to the following series: n-pentane → ethanol → water.
e. Both a and c are true.

59. Liquid water ...

a. at a pressure of 1 atm, has its maximum density at the temperature of 3.8°C
b. at a pressure of 1 atm, has its maximum density at the temperature of 0°C
c. at a pressure of 1 atm, has its maximum density at the temperature of 100°C
d. at a pressure of 1 atm, has a minimum density at the temperature of 98°C
e. at a pressure of 1 atm, a presión de 1 atm, has a minimum density of 0.89 kg/l, at 100°C

60. Which of the following sentences is FALSE? On Earth...

a. There is more fresh water below the surface than in atmosphere.
b. There is more water in atmosphere than in rivers.
c. Below the surface, there is more salt water than fresh water.
d. There is more salt water in oceans and seas than fresh water frozen in the polar ice-caps and continental glaciers.
e. There is more water in rivers, reservoirs and lakes, than in continental glaciers and permafrost.

61. Van't Hoff's equation calculates the value of osmotic pressure as a function of some characteristics of solute, its concentration and temperature. In this context, which of the following sentences is TRUE?

a. The higher the temperature, the higher the osmotic pressure.
b. The higher the osmolarity, the higher the osmotic pressure.
c. The higher the solute concentration, the higher the osmotic pressure.
d. a, b and c are true.
e. a is false, b and c are true.

62. Osmosis ...

a. is a physical phenomenon that determines that, between two solutions sepparated by a semipermeable membrane, solvent moves from the hipertonic to the hipotonic medium.

b. is a physical phenomenon that determines that, between two solutions sepparated by a semipermeable membrane, solvent moves from the hipotonic to the hipertonic medium.

c. is a physical phenomenon that determines that, between two solutions sepparated by a permeable membrane, solvent moves from the hipertonic to the hipotonic medium.

d. is a physical phenomenon that determines that, between two solutions sepparated by a permeable membrane, solvent moves from the hipotonic to the hipertonic medium.

e. is a physical phenomenon that determines that, between two solutions sepparated by a semipermeable membrane, solute moves from the hipertonic to the hipotonic medium.

63. Van't Hoff's factor...

a. is the magnitude that indicates the solubility of a salt.

b. is a parameter that indicates the amount of chemical species that arise from a solute after dissolving it within a given solvent.

c. is a parameter that indicates the difference in osmolarity associated to the same solute at two different given temperatures (T_a and T_b).

d. is a parameter that indicates the rate of change in the osmolarity of a chemical specie when it duplicates its concentratiion at constant temperature.

e. is a constant proporcionality factor ($i = 0.73$ $N \cdot M^{-1}$) that multiplies concentration, temperature and gas constant in van't Hoff's equation for calculating osmotic pressure.

64. We extract lysosomes from a cell culture of hepatocytes, and we conserve them in a glucose solution. The concentration of NaCl and KCl in these organelles is 0.1 M and 0.05 M, respectively. Knowing that both salts have a van't Hoff's factor of 2, what should be glucose concentration for the changes in lysosomes volume, due to osmosis, to be minimum? NOTE: glucose van't Hoff's factor is 1.

a. 0.075 M
b. 0.150 M
c. 0.225 M
d. 0.300 M
e. 0.375 M

Carbohydrates

65. We can define 'carbohydrates' as 'those molecules with stoichometric formula _____ or those chemically derived from them'. Which is this stoichometric formula?

  a. $(C_2HO)_n$
  b. $(CH)_n$
  c. $(CHO)_n$
  d. $(CH_2O)_n$
  e. $(C_2H_4O)_n$

66. Which of the following molecules, shown as Fisher's projection, corresponds to D-glucose?

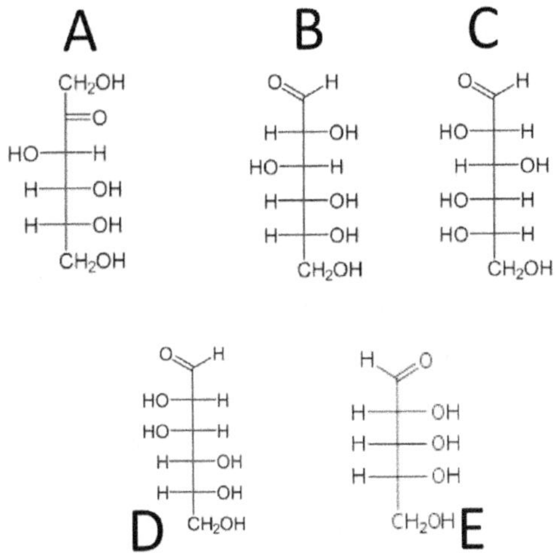

  a. A
  b. B
  c. C
  d. D
  e. E

67. Which of the following sentences is FALSE?

  a. Glyceraldehyde and dihydroxyacetone are tautomers.
  b. Two enantiomers are molecules that structurally are non-superposable mirror images one of the other.
  c. Glyceraldehhyde can be as two enantiomers, known as forms D and L.
  d. If we have, in a solution, only the D forms of given monosacharyde, this solution will deviate the polarized light plane to the right.
  e. A solution of L-glyceraldehyde will deviate the polarized light plane to the left.

68. Which of the following molecules, shown as Fisher's projections, corresponds to D-fructose?

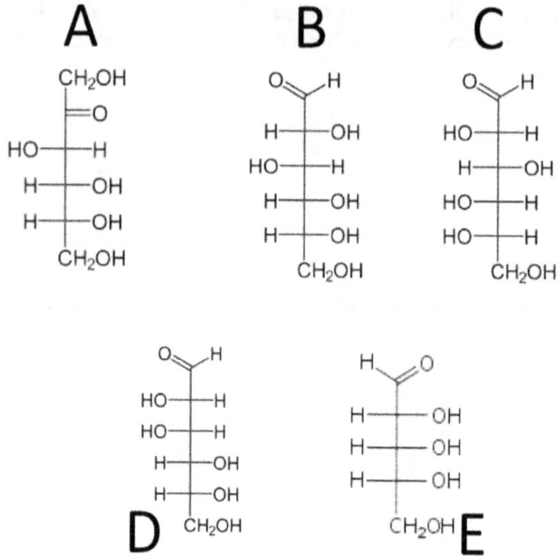

a. A
b. B
c. C
d. D
e. E

69. There is a glucoseminoglycan highly sulfated (with three sulfate groups for each monosaccharide that compose it) that, by its binding to antiprothrombin-III, inhibits blood coagulation process. It is...

a. ...chondroitin sulfate
b. ...heparin
c. ...heparan sulfate
d. ...hyaluronic acid
e. ...dermatan sulfate

70. What is the proper way of naming this disaccharide?

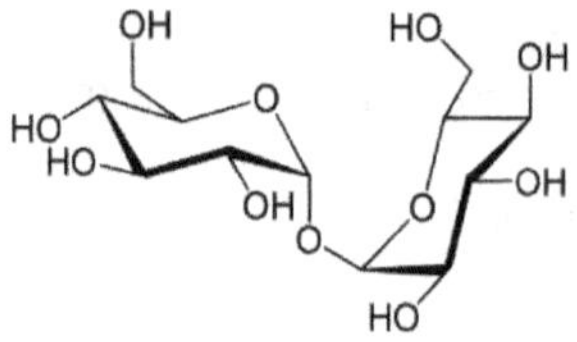

a. β-D-glucopyranosyl(1→6)β-D-glucopyranose
b. β-D-galactopiranosil(1→4)β-D-glucopyranose
c. β-D-glucopiranosyl(1→4)β-D-glucopyranose
d. α-D-glucopiranosyl(1→2)β-D-fructofuranoside
e. α-D-glucopiranosyl(1→1)α-D-glucopyranose

71. Which of the following sentences is FALSE?

a. The most abundant forms of natural monosacharydes are D forms.
b. A glucose molecule has 6 carbon atoms.
c. Tetroses have the following empirical formula: $(CH_2O)_4$.
d. An aldotetrose has two chiral centers, thus it has 4 possible stereoisomers.
e. In no-cyclic monosacharydes, the nomenclature D and L refers to the configuration of the chiral carbon which is nearest to carbonile group.

72. Which of the following molecules, shown as Fisher's projections, corresponds to D-mannose?

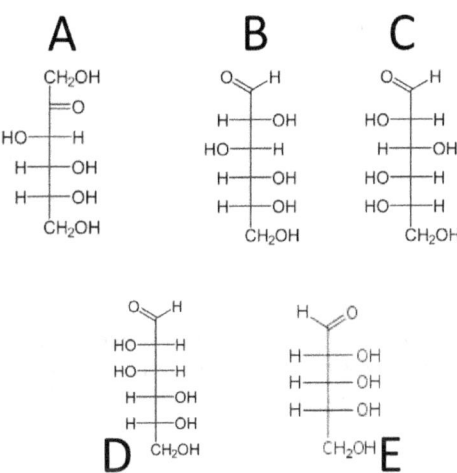

a. A
b. B
c. C
d. D
e. E

73. Which of the following molecules are glycosides?

a. ouabain
b. muramic acid
c. amygdalin
d. erythritol
e. a and c are TRUE

74. Which of the following molecules is a glycoside?

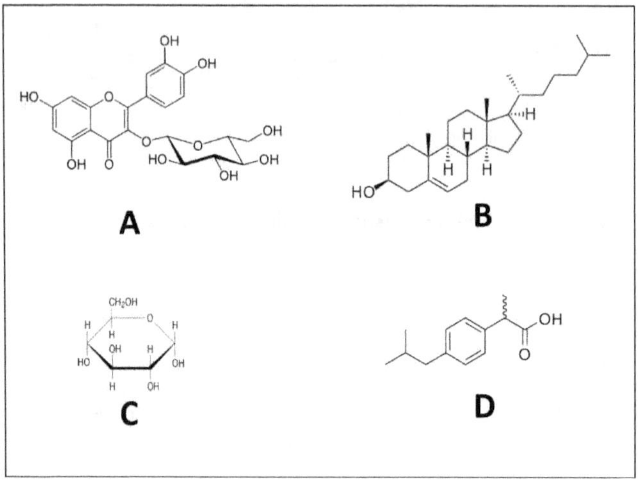

A

B

C

D

a. A
b. B
c. C
d. D
e. B and D

75. Among the following molecules, there is a glycoside which is characteristic since ancient tribes around Somalia use it as a poison for darts. It is an inhibitor of Na+/K+ pump and is currently used as drug for some heart disfunctions. Which is this molecule?

a. amygdalin
b. ouabain
c. trehalose
d. mannitol
e. sorbitol

76. Which of the following molecules, shown as Fisher's projections, does correspond to L-glucose?

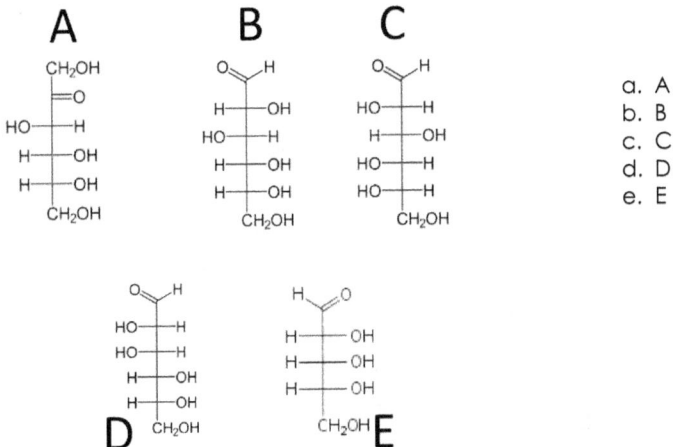

a. A
b. B
c. C
d. D
e. E

77. Which of the following molecules does correspond to dihydroxyacetone?

A   B   C

a. A
b. B
c. C
d. D
e. E

D   E

78. Which of the following molecules does correspond to the monomer that constitutes the basic unit of chitin?

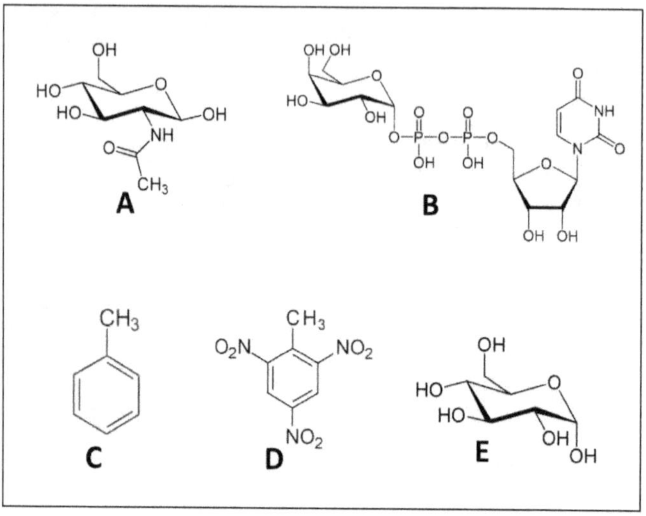

a. A
b. B
c. C
d. D
e. E

79. Sucrose is a disaccharide formed by the union of ...

a. 2 α-D-glucoses by an O-glycosidic (1→4) bond
b. 2 β-D-glucoses by an O-glycosidic (1→4) bond
c. 2 β-D-glucoses by an O-glycosidic (1→6) bond
d. β-D-galactose and β-D-glucose by an O-glycosidic (1→4) bond
e. α-D-glucose and β-D-fructose by an O-glycosidic (1→2) bond

80. Which is the proper way of naming this disaccharide?

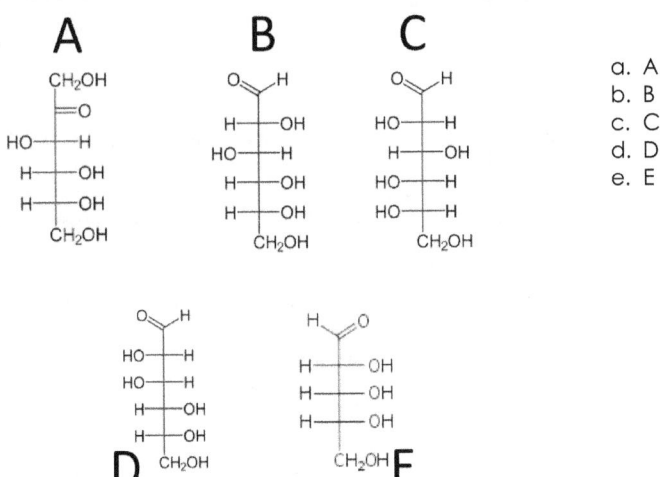

a. β-D-glucopyranosyl(1→6)β-D-glucopyranose
b. β-D-galactopyranosyl(1→4)β-D-glucopyranose
c. β-D-glucopyranosyl(1→4)β-D-glucopyranose
d. α-D-glucopyranosyl(1→2)β-D-fructofuranoside
e. α-D-glucopyranosyl(1→1)α-D-glucopyranose

81. Which of the following molecules, shown as Fisher's projections, does correspond to D-ribose?

a. A
b. B
c. C
d. D
e. E

82. Which of the following molecules is a monosaccharide?

a. lactose
b. maltose
c. galactose
d. cellobiose
e. starch

83. Which of the following sentences is FALSE?

a. Mutarotase enzymes catalyze interconversion between α and β forms of a cyclic monosaccharide.
b. Cyclic forms (of furanose and pyranose type) of monosaccharides in solution adopt preferably plane structures.
c. In the cyclic form of α-D-glucopyranose, the chair configuration is more stable than the boat configuration.
d. Any cyclic monosaccharide with a pyranose structure will preferably adopt, in aqueos solution, the conformation in which the number of voluminous substituents (-OH) in equatorial position would be maximized.
e. α-D-sedoheptulopyranose presents a cycic structure with hexagonal form, preferably in boat conformation.

84. β-D-glucopyranose in chair conformation and β-D-glucopyranose in boat conformation are...

a. cyclic pentagonal structures in which the ring is formed by 4 carbons and 1 oxygen
b. linear aldohexoses
c. molecules with the same stereochemical configuration but that differ in its tridimensional conformation
d. cyclic hexagonal structures in which the ring is formed by 6 carbons
e. two forms of glucose that are configurational isomers

85. Which of the following molecules is erythrulose?

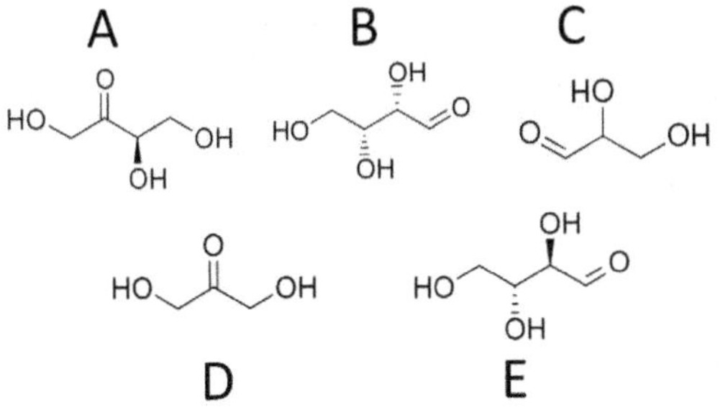

a. A
b. B
c. C
d. D
e. E

86. Which of the following sentences is FALSE?

a. Under physiological conditions, phosphate esters of natural monosaccharides are found as a mixture of monoanions and dianions.
b. Soft oxidation of β-D-glucopyranose with Cu(II) in a basic environment (Fehling solution) produces D-gluconic acid, Cu_2O and water.
c. Under physiological conditions, the D-gluconic acid present in solution is in equilibrium with the D-δ-gluconolactone.
d. The generation of a red precipitate (Cu_2O) coming from oxidation of monosaccharides, is a classical proof for detecting free sugars, and has been historically employed in urine analysis for diabetes detection.
e. The reduction of the carbonil group of a natural monosaccharide produces alditols (like erythritol, D-mannitol, sorbitol,...).

87. Among the following disaccharides, one of them is characteristic because, as it has no free hemiacetalyc carbons, it has not reducing power. Which is it?

a. maltose
b. lactose
c. cellobiose
d. trehalose
e. sucrose

88. Which of the following molecules is threose?

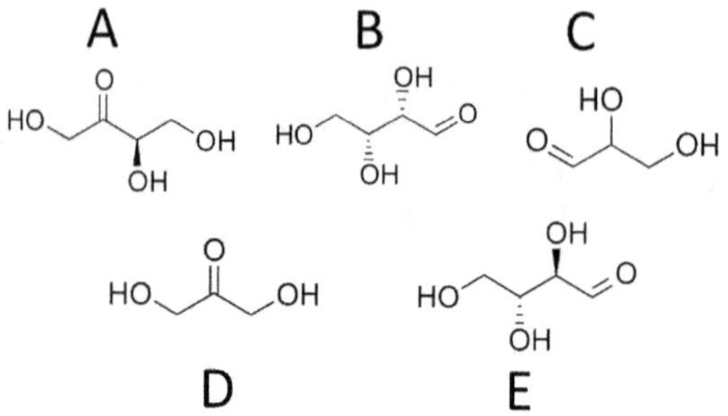

a. A
b. B
c. C
d. D
e. E

89. Maltose is a disaccharide formed by the bonding of...

a. 2 α-D-glucoses by an O-glycosidic (1→4) bond
b. 2 β-D-glucoses by an O-glycosidic (1→4) bond
c. 2 β-D-glucoses by an O-glycosidic (1→6) bond
d. β-D-galactose and β-D-glucose by an O-glycosidic (1→4) bond
e. α-D-glucose and β-D-fructose by an O-glycosidic (1→2) bond

90. Glucose is a...

a. triose
b. tetrose
c. pentose
d. hexose
e. heptose

91. An alditol...

a. is formed by the oxidation of sugars, as it occurs in Fehling's reaction
b. is formed by the reduction of the carbonil of a monosaccharide
c. is formed by the reaction of ketohexoses with Ag^+, as it occurs in Tollens' reaction
d. is a molecule as for example amygdalin
e. is an amino derivative of a natural monosaccharide

92. Which of the following molecules is erythrose?

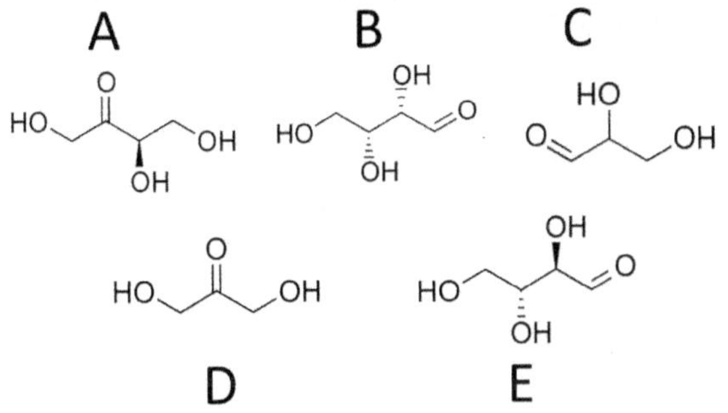

a. A
b. B
c. C
d. D
e. E

93. Which is the proper way of naming this disaccharide?

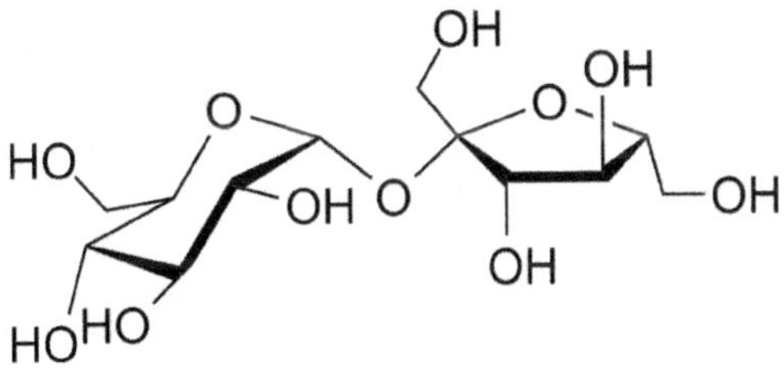

a. β-D-glucopyranosyl(1→6)β-D-glucopyranose
b. β-D-galactopyranosyl(1→4)β-D-glucopyranose
c. β-D-glucopyranosyl(1→4)β-D-glucopyranose
d. α-D-glucopyranosyl(1→2)β-D-fructofuranoside
e. α-D-glucopyranosyl(1→1)α-D-glucopyranose

94. Cataracts that are frequently formed in the crystalline lens of diabetic people are accumulations of a derivative of natural monosaccarides named...

    a. muramic acid
    b. gluconic acid
    c. sialic acid
    d. mannitol
    e. sorbitol

95. Imagine an oligosaccharide with the following sequence (glucose-lyxose-xylose-arabinose-fructose). What would be the proper way of writting it by using the 3-letters abreviatted codes for each monosaccharide?

    a. Glu-Lix-Xil-Ara-Fru
    b. Glc-Lyx-Xyl-Ara-Fru
    c. Glc-Lyx-Xyl-Arb-Frc
    d. Glc-Lix-Xyl-Ara-Fru
    e. Glu-Lyx-Xyl-Ara-Frc

96. Bacteria can be classified as Gram positive or Gram negative. Ths differenciation is based in the behaviour of bacteria in a Gram staining procedure, that also depends on the presence of exposed peptidoglycanes in bacterial wall. Thus...

    a. ... Gram positive bacteria have only one layer of peptidoglycanes, recovered by a lipid bilayer, that absorbs colouring in Gram's staining
    b. ... Gram negative bacteria have many layers of peptidoglycanes, where colouring of Gram's staining is retained
    c. ... Gram positive bacteria have many layers of peptidoglycanes, where colouring of Gram's staining is retained
    d. ... Gram negative bacteria have many layers of peptidoglycanes, that repel colouring of Gram's staining
    e. a and d are true

97. Which of the following schemes or molecular formulas does correpond to a lipoteichoic acid, that we find in the membrane of some bacteria?

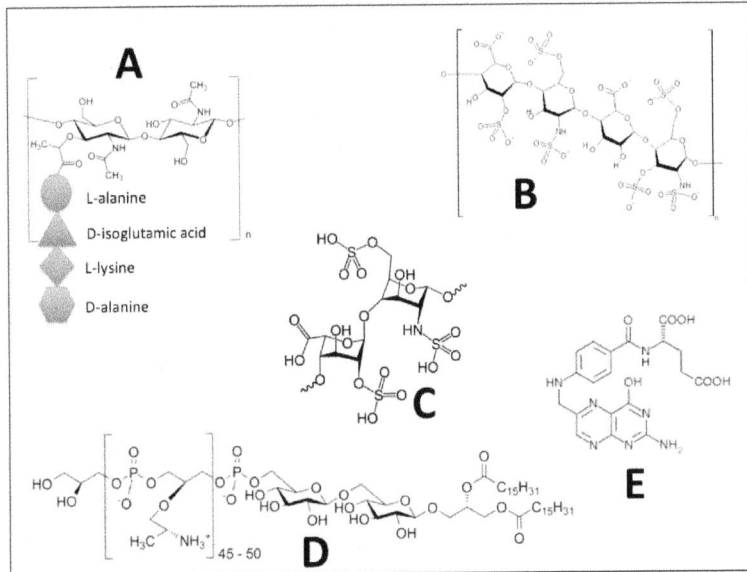

a. A
b. B
c. C
d. D
e. E

98. Ribulose is a...

a. triose
b. tetrose
c. pentose
d. hexose
e. heptose

99. Which of the following molecules is glyceraldehyde?

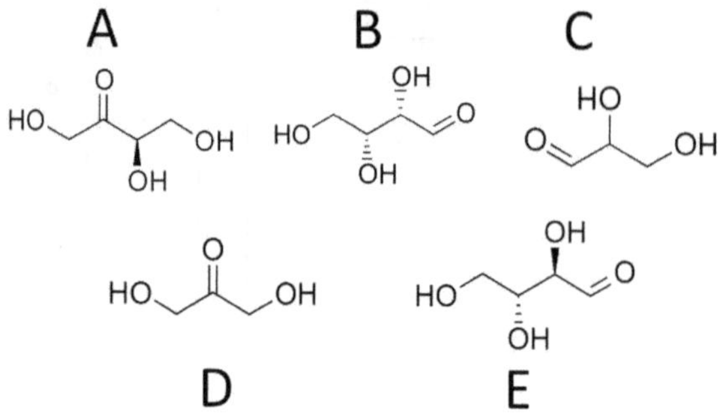

a. A
b. B
c. C
d. D
e. E

100. Which of the following polysaccharides is 'the most abundant polymer in Biosphere'?

a. cellulose
b. glycogen
c. starch
d. chitin
e. chondroitin sulfate

101. Sorbose is a...

a. triose
b. tetrose
c. pentose
d. hexose
e. heptose

102. Gentiobiose is a disacharyde formed by the bonding of...

a. 2 α-D-glucoses by an O-glycosidic (1→4) bond
b. 2 β-D-glucoses by an O-glycosidic (1→4) bond
c. 2 β-D-glucoses by an O-glycosidic (1→6) bond
d. β-D-galactose and β-D-glucose by an O-glycosidic (1→4) bond
e. α-D-glucose and β-D-fructose by an O-glycosidic (1→2) bond

103. Cellulose is....

a. a polymer of D-glucose
b. a polymer of monosaccharides bound by $\beta(1\rightarrow4)$ bonds
c. a polymer in which each D-glucose presents a turn of ~180° from the previous residue
d. a and b are true, c is false
e. a, b and c are true

104. Dihydroxyacetone is a...

a. triose
b. tetrose
c. pentose
d. hexose
e. heptose

105. Human body contains enzymes that can metabolize starch. They are amylases and are unable to break cellulose. Which of the differences between starch and cellulose could account for this behaviour?

a. starch is made by fructoses and cellulose by glucoses
b. starch is made by glucoses and cellulose by fructoses
c. in starch, glucoses are linked by means of $\alpha(1\rightarrow4)$ bonds, and in cellulose they are linked by means of $\beta(1\rightarrow4)$ bonds
d. in starch, glucoses are linked by means of $\beta(1\rightarrow4)$ bonds, and in cellulose they are linked by means of $\alpha(1\rightarrow4)$ bonds
e. cellulose presents many ramifications, that are absent in starch, and difficult access of amylases to O-glycosidic bonds

106. Which of the following disaccharides are not a reducing agent, and thus would give negative result in a Fehling's test?

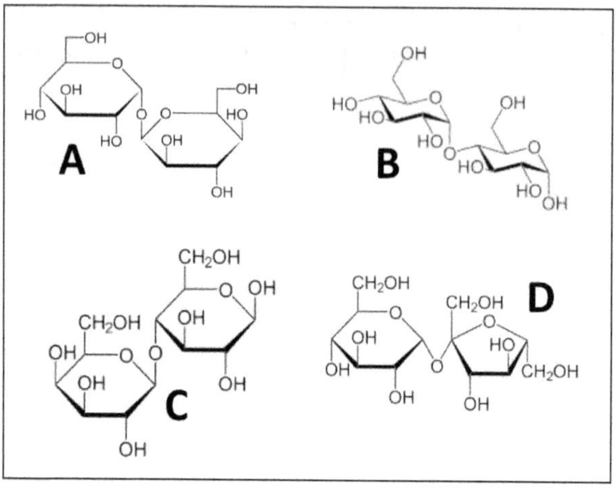

a. C and B
b. A and C
c. A and D
d. B and D
e. A and B

107. Glyceraldehyde is a...

a. triose
b. tetrose
c. pentose
d. hexose
e. heptose

108. Which is the proper way of naming the following disaccharide?

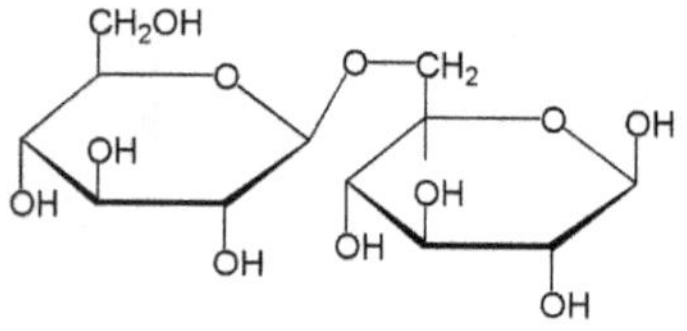

a. β-D-glucopyranosyl(1→6)β-D-glucopyranose
b. β-D-galactopyranosyl(1→4)β-D-glucopyranose
c. β-D-glucopyranosyl(1→4)β-D-glucopyranose
d. α-D-glucopyranosyl(1→2)β-D-fructofuranoside
e. α-D-glucopyranosyl(1→1)α-D-glucopyranose

109. Many "sugar free" chewing gums are really sweetened with sorbitol, that is less energetic than sucrose or starch, since it only produces 2,4 cal/g, compared to the ~4 cal/g produced by them. Sorbitol is...

a. a derivative produced by amination of glucose
b. a derivative produced by oxidation of glucose
c. a derivative produced by reduction of glucose
d. a derivative produced by the formation of an O-glycosydic bond, with the loss of a water molecule, between glucose and an aromatic residue very similar to phenol
e. a derivative produced by phosphorilation of glucose

110. Erythrulose is a...

a. triose
b. tetrose
c. pentose
d. hexose
e. heptose

111. To name some deriivatives of natural monosacharydes, we use an standard nomeclature, generally in accordance with the english name of the molecule. By applying this nomenclature, which of the following relationships is wrong?

a. GlcN → N-acetyl glucose
b. GlcUA → glucuronic acid
c. GalN → galactosamine
d. GlcNAc → N-acetylglucosamina
e. NeuNAc → N-acetylneuraminic acid

112. Threose is a ...

a. triose
b. tetrose
c. pentose
d. hexose
e. heptose

113. Hemicellulose...

a. is a type of cellulose of fungic origin that can be metabolized by human digestive enzymes, so being employed, with alginates, gels and other derivatives in food industry
b. is a term used to name a group of complex polysacharydes, among which we find xylanes and glucomannanes, usually found in the woody stalks of many plants
c. is a form of cellulose, in which the O-glycosydic bonds between consecutive glucoses are not of ~180° but approximately the half (in a range from 80° to 100°)
d. is an heteropolysaccharide similar to cellulose, where approximately half the D-glucoses have been substituted by other monosaccharides, very often galactose, although not exclusively
e. is a cellulose derivative where interchain bonds are of a lower intensity, giving rise to complexes of lower size. It was originally detected in polymers with a molecular weight of approximately the 50% of the molecular weight of celllulose, so the use of the hemi- prefix in their original name

114. Which of the following sentences is FALSE?

a. Cellulose is found in animal kingdom in the stiff external mantle of some tunicates
b. Cellulose has been found in human connective tissue
c. Cellulose, as an structural support substance, has been mainly given up during animal evolution
d. Fungi often use, as an structural supprot agent, homopolysacharides of glucose (glucans) similar to cellulose, although they have $\beta(1{\rightarrow}3)$ bonds instead of $\beta(1{\rightarrow}6)$ ones
e. Cellulose has been found, with a relatively high abundance (~1%), in corneous structures like baleens

115. Which of the following schemes or molecular formulas does correspond to heparine, that is a glycosaminoglucan used as an anticoagulant drug?

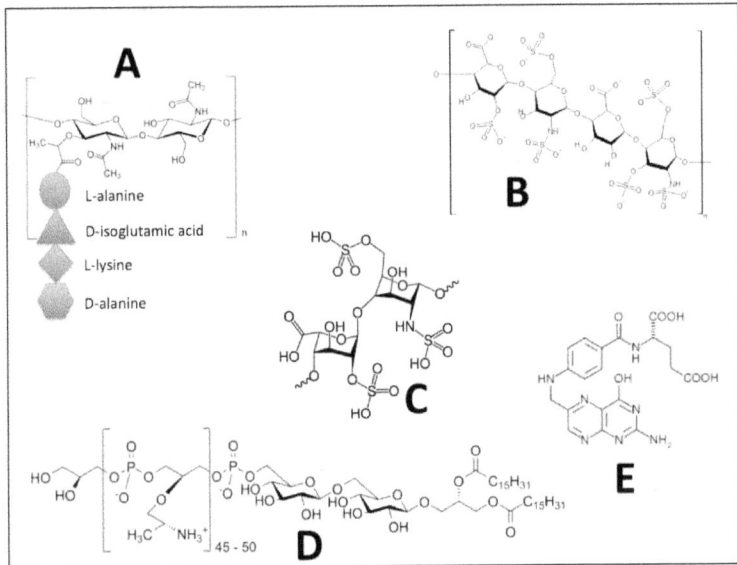

a. A
b. B
c. C
d. D
e. E

116. Ocassionally, in proteoglycans, two long polysaccharide chains are bound by a covalent bridge in which a curious chemical element participates. These unions are quite frequent, around 1 for each 100 monosaccharides. What is this element?

a. silicon
b. nickel
c. lithium
d. calcium
e. cobalt

117. Tagatose is a ...

a. triose
b. tetrose
c. pentose
d. hexose
e. heptose

118. O-glycosidic bond formation between two monosaccharides to form a disaccharide causes the net release...

a. of a proton
b. of an O_2 molecule
c. of a H_2 molecule
d. of two protons
e. of a water molecule

119. Under physiological conditions, hydrolysis of a standard disaccharide (i.e. lactose)...

a. is favoured by a standard Gibbs free energy of ~2 kJ/mol
b. is favoured by a standard Gibbs free energy of ~15 kJ/mol
c. is disfavoured by a standard Gibbs free energy of ~2 kJ/mol
d. is disfavoured by a standard Gibbs free energy of ~15 kJ/mol
e. is disfavoured by a standard Gibbs free energy of ~150 kJ/mol

120. Hydrolysis of polysaccharides under physiological conditions...

a. is spontaneous and fast
b. requires enzymatic catalysis to achieve a speed suitable for almost all physiological requirements
c. is thermodynamically unfavourable
d. cannot occur at a speed suitable for almost all physiological requirements, since it would need pH values near 12
e. is clearly unfavoured (in terms of free energy) when it comes both to kinetics and thermodynamics

121. Which of the following polysaccharides IS NOT, in general terms, a polysaccharide for energy storage?

a. Amylose
b. Amylopectin
c. Glycogen
d. Chitin
e. All of them are polysaccharides essentially employed for energy storage

122. In which of the following tissues or materials would we find the highest concentration of glycogen?

a. Mammal liver
b. Potato starch
c. Mammal dermis
d. Mammal bone matrix
e. Phloem

123. In which of the following tissues or materials would we find the highest concentration of starch?

a. Mammal liver
b. Xylem
c. Coconut milk
d. Adenoid glands
e. Rice

124. Amylose, Glycogen and amylopectin are polymers of...

a. β-D-glucopyranose
b. α-D-glucopyranose
c. β-D-fructofuranose
d. α-D-fructofuranose
e. β-D-galactopyranose

125. Amylose...

a. ...is a linear polymer constituted by glucoses connected by α(1→2) bonds
b. ... is a linear polymer constituted by glucoses connected by α(1→3) bonds
c. ... is a linear polymer constituted by glucoses connected by α(1→4) bonds
d. ... is a linear polymer constituted by glucoses connected by α(1→5) bonds
e. ... is a linear polymer constituted by glucoses connected by α(1→6) bonds

126. Amylopectin...

a. ...is a ramified polymer constituted by glucoses connected by $\alpha(1\rightarrow2)$ and $\alpha(1\rightarrow4)$ bonds
b. ...is a ramified polymer constituted by glucoses connected by $\alpha(1\rightarrow6)$ and $\alpha(1\rightarrow4)$ bonds
c. ...is a ramified polymer constituted by glucoses connected by $\alpha(1\rightarrow4)$ and $\beta(1\rightarrow4)$ bonds
d. ...is a ramified polymer constituted by glucoses connected by $\alpha(1\rightarrow2)$ and $\beta(1\rightarrow6)$ bonds
e. ...is a ramified polymer constituted by glucoses connected by $\alpha(4\rightarrow6)$ and $\alpha(4\rightarrow4)$ bonds

127. Glycogen...

a. ...is a ramified polymer constituted by glucoses connected by $\alpha(1\rightarrow2)$ and $\alpha(1\rightarrow4)$ bonds
b. ...is a ramified polymer constituted by glucoses connected by $\alpha(1\rightarrow6)$ and $\alpha(1\rightarrow4)$ bonds
c. ...is a ramified polymer constituted by glucoses connected by $\alpha(1\rightarrow4)$ and $\beta(1\rightarrow4)$ bonds
d. ...is a ramified polymer constituted by glucoses connected by $\alpha(1\rightarrow2)$ and $\beta(1\rightarrow6)$ bonds
e. ...is a ramified polymer constituted by glucoses connected by $\alpha(4\rightarrow6)$ and $\alpha(4\rightarrow4)$ bonds

128. Which of the following sentences is FALSE?

a. Glycogen is a polymer more ramified than amylose
b. Glycogen is a polymer more ramified than amylopectin
c. The release of free glucose is faster from glycogen than from starch
d. The branches, due to $\alpha(1\rightarrow6)$ bonds between glucoses, appear approximately each 8-12 glucoses in amylopectin
e. Amylose is a linear polymer

129. Amylose is a linear polymer, with helicoidal structure, in which we find...

a. ... 4 glucoses for each helix turn
b. ... 6 glucoses for each helix turn
c. ... 8 glucoses for each helix turn
d. ... 10 glucoses for each helix turn
e. ... 12 glucoses for each helix turn

130. Polymerization of monosaccharides to form big molecules inside the cell confers, to those cells that are able to do it, the following adaptative feature...

a. It avoids sharp variations in intracellular osmotic pressure
b. It allows to regulate the flux of generation of soluble monosaccharides by controlling gene expression
c. It allows the intake of extracellular monosaccharides, even if it is done against a concentration gradient
d. It allows to store more monosaccharides in less space
e. All the previous sentences are TRUE

131. Which of the following molecules IS NOT a glycosaminoglycan?

a. Hyaluronic acid
b. Chondroitin sulfate
c. Dermatan sulfate
d. Heparin
e. Sialic acid

132. Which of the following schemes or molecular formulas does correspond to peptidoglycan that we find in Gram positive bacteria?

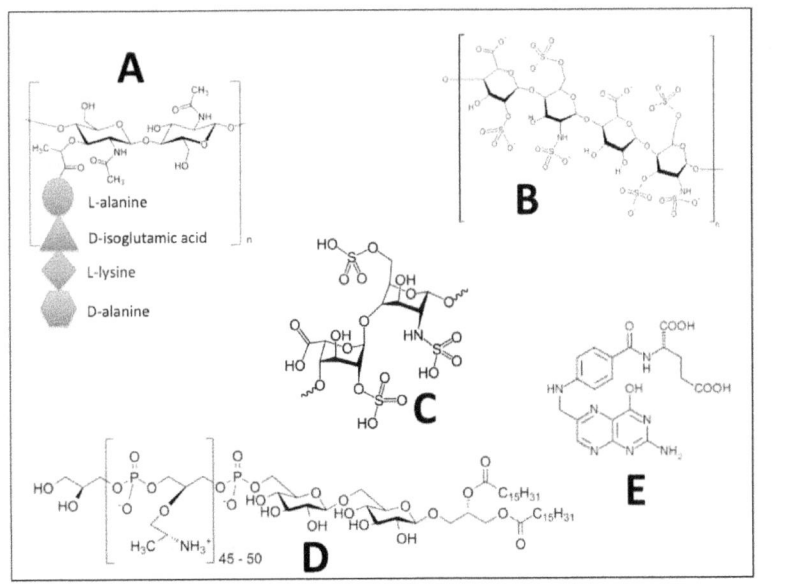

a. A
b. B
c. C
d. D
e. E

133. Psicose is a ...

a. triose
b. tetrose
c. pentose
d. hexose
e. heptose

134. There is a polysaccharide of natural origin which basic repetitive unit can be symbolized as GlcUAβ(1→3)GlcNAc. We also know that these disaccharide subunits are connected by β(1→4) bonds. Which is this polysacharide?

a. starch
b. murein
c. glycogen
d. heparan sulfate
e. hyaluronic acid

135. Erythrose is a...

a. triose
b. tetrose
c. pentose
d. hexose
e. heptose

136. Talose is a...

a. triose
b. tetrose
c. pentose
d. hexose
e. heptose

137. Which is the proper way of naming the following disaccharide?

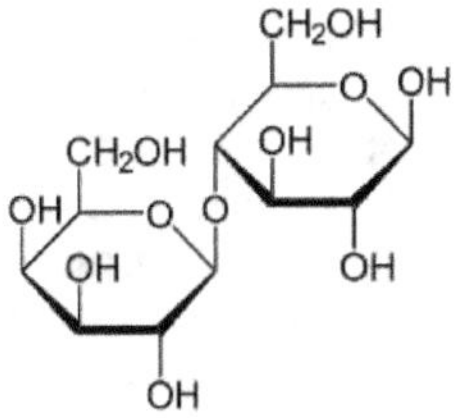

a. β-D-glucopyranosyl(1→6)β-D-glucopyranose
b. β-D-galactopyranosyl(1→4)β-D-glucopyranose
c. β-D-glucopyranosyl(1→4)β-D-glucopyranose
d. α-D-glucopyranosyl(1→2)β-D-fructofuranoside
e. α-D-glucopyranosyl(1→1)α-D-glucopyranose

138. Sedoheptulose is a...

a. triose
b. tetrose
c. pentose
d. hexose
e. heptose

139. The antigens responsible for human blood types (ABO) are a group of oligosaccharides linked to proteins and/or lipids of plasma membrane of red blood cells. When it comes to these antigens, which of the following sentences is FALSE?

a. each antigen of group A contains a fucose, a galactose, two residues of N-acetylgalactosamine and one of sialic acid
b. each antigen of B group contains, at least, a galactose
c. each antigen of group 0 contains sialic acid and, at least, a fucose
d. each antigen of 0 group contains two residues of N-acetylgalactosamine
e. all the antigens of ABO system are anchored to the membrane by means of a residue of N-acetylgalactosamine

140. Arabinose is a...

a. triose
b. tetrose
c. pentose
d. hexose
e. heptose

141. We can roughly assume that, during evolution, when organisms acquired certain sizes, it began to be beneficial, when it comes to biological efficiency, the development of structures for mechanical support (skeletons). el desarrollo de estructuras de soporte mecánico (esqueletos). In different groups of living beings, different strategies prevailed. In vertebrates, internal skeletons, based on mineralization on a basal matrix of _____ were developed. Annelides chose exoskeletons formed by matter crystallized on a matrix of _____. In arthropods, the most succesful strategy was building exoskeletons by mineralization on a matrix of _____.

    a. collagen / calcium carbonate / collagen
    b. hydroxylapatite / collagen / chitin
    c. collagen / collagen / chitin
    d. calcium carbonate / ketamine / chitin
    e. collagen / calcium carbonate / chitin

142. Glycosaminoglycans are...

    a. oligosaccharides of glucosamina
    b. heteropolysaccharides with net positive charge
    c. homopolysaccharides with net positive charge
    d. heteropolysaccharides with net negative charge
    e. homopolysaccharides with net negative charge

143. Altrose is a...

    a. triose
    b. tetrose
    c. pentose
    d. hexose
    e. heptose

144. Xylulose is a...

    a. triose
    b. tetrose
    c. pentose
    d. hexose
    e. heptose

145. Mannoheptulose is a...

a. triose
b. tetrose
c. pentose
d. hexose
e. heptose

146. To name some deriivatives of natural monosacharydes, we use an standard nomeclature, generally in accordance with the english name of the molecule. By applying this nomenclature, which of the following relationships is wrong?

a. GlcA → gluconic acid
b. GlcUA → glucuronic acid
c. GalN → galactosamine
d. GalNAc → N-acetylgalactosamine
e. NeuNAc → N-acetylneubruphene

147. Which of the following schemes or chemical formulas does correspond to the glycosaminoglycan called heparan sulfate?

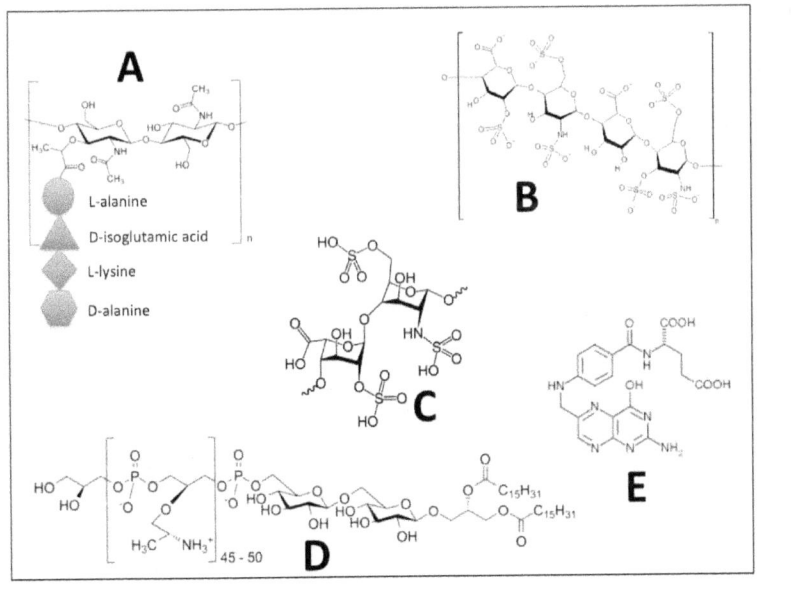

a. A
b. B
c. C
d. D
e. E

148. Psicose is a...

a. triose
b. tetrose
c. pentose
d. hexose
e. heptose

149. Cellobiose is a disaccharide formed by the union of...

a. 2 α-D-glucoses by means of a (1→4) glycosidic bond
b. 2 β-D-glucoses by means of a (1→4) glycosidic bond
c. 2 β-D-glucoses by means of a (1→6) glycosidic bond
d. β-D-galactose and β-D-glucose by means of a (1→4) glycosidic bond
e. α-D-glucose and β-D-fructose by means of a (1→2) glycosidic bond

150. Idose is a...

a. triose
b. tetrose
c. pentose
d. hexose
e. heptose

151. Which of the following disaccharides are reducing agents and, thus, would give a positive result in a Fehling's test?

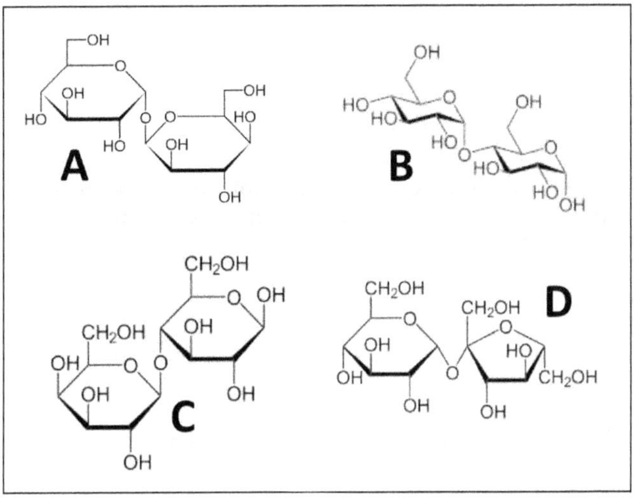

a. C and B
b. A and C
c. A and D
d. B and D
e. A and B

152. Gulose is a...

a. triose
b. tetrose
c. pentose
d. hexose
e. heptose

153. Which of the following sentences is TRUE?

a. Chitin is found in the septum formed between two yeast dividing cells
b. Chitin has been found in some fungi
c. Chitin has been found in some algae
d. Chitin is specially abundant in exoskeleton of arthropods
e. All are TRUE

154. Galactose is a...

a. triose
b. tetrose
c. pentose
d. hexose
e. heptose

155. A solution of α-D-galactopyranogalactose causes a rotation in the plane of polarized light. If this solution is treated with a reducing agent, such property is lost. What is the molecular cause of this behaviour?

a. α-D-galactopiranose is broken into two trioses
b. chiral carbons of α-D-galactopiranose loss chirality
c. α-D-galactopiranose polymerizes forming chains similar to those of amylose, with bonds α(1→4)
d. α-D-galactopiranose is transformed into CO_2 and water
e. α-D-galactopiranose polymerizes forming chains similar to those of amylose, with bonds β(1→4)

156. Lactose is a disaccharide formed by the union of...

a. 2 α-D-glucoses by means of a (1→4) glycosidic bond
b. 2 β-D-glucoses by means of a (1→4) glycosidic bond
c. 2 β-D-glucoses by means of a (1→6) glycosidic bond
d. β-D-galactose and β-D-glucose by means of a (1→4) glycosidic bond
e. α-D-glucose and β-D-fructose by means of a (1→2) glycosidic bond

157. Where does the term 'racemic' come from? It is employed to refer to solutions of chiral molecules where the proportion of each enantiomer is around 50%.

a. In texts attributed to Babylonian science, the term 'raknnus' is employed to refer to mixtures. This term was adapted by Pasteur when he discovered the optical activity of para-tartaric acid, naming 'recemic' to the mixtures without optical activity.

b. In the deposites accumulated in wine bottles, there was found para tartaric acid, also named racemic acid (from latin: *racemus*, bunch of grapes). This compund was that crystallized by Pasteur to later sepparate crystals with opposed optical activity.

c. Pasteur did not employed the terminology 'racemic' to refer to mixtures of compounds, but it was London Royal Society that coined the term at the end of 19th century. Since chromatographies, called 'races' in the jargon of british scientists, were employed to sepparate enantiomers, the mixture of compounds participating in such experiments began to be named 'race mixture' in some papers, finally diverting into the adjective 'racemic', early standarized by the stated institution.

d. The term comes from latin: *racemis*, mixture, set of provissions. In some Romance languages we find words with the same root (rebost, racomat, reossi...)

e. In the first experiments to demonstrate the opposite optical activity between crystals of high enantiomeric purity, done with p-tartaric acid, Pasteur did not use the term 'racemic'. A few years later, he found that this phenomenon of enantiomeric sepparation is particularly difficult to achieve with the 'racemic acid' (one of the many phenolic compounds present in wine) and then started to name 'racemic' to the mixtures of enantiomers.

158. Chitin is a polysaccharide formed by units of...

a. α-D-glucose
b. N-methyl-α-D-fructose
c. acetylsalicylic acid
d. N-acetyl-β-D-glucosamina
e. sialic acid

159. Among the following molecules there is a glycoside unique by its smell of bitter almonds, which is?

a. amygdalin
b. ouabain
c. trehalose
d. mannitol
e. sorbitol

160. The following figure represents α-D-glucopyranose in chair conformation, which of the chiral carbons have the OH groups in equatorial position?

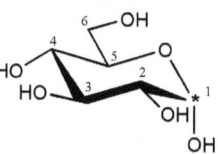

a. 1, 2, 3 and 4
b. 1, 2 and 3
c. 1 and 2
d. 2, 3 and 4
e. none of the options is true

161. Glucidic residues that bind to proteins by N- type bonds, bind residues of ...

a. serine
b. threonine
c. methionine
d. asparagine
e. phenylalanine

162. Oligosaccharydes that bind proteins by N- type bonds normally use, as monosaccharides to bind asparagin,...

a. glucose or N-acetylglucose
b. N-acetylglucosamina or N-acetylgalactosamine
c. mannose or trehalose
d. mannitol or sorbitol
e. N-acetylpyridine or N-methylglucosamina

163. Oligosaccharides that bind proteins by a bond of O- type use to form a bond between _____ and the OH group of _____ or _____.

    a. N-acetylgalactosamine / threonine / serine
    b. galactosamine / phenylalanine / tyrosine
    c. N-methylglucosamina / phenylalanine / tyrosine
    d. glucosamina / threonine / serine
    e. N-methylglucosamina / threonine / serine

164. The antigens responsible for human blood types (ABO) are a group of oligosaccharides linked to proteins and/or lipids of plasma membrane of red blood cells. When it comes to these antigens, which of the following sentences is FALSE?

    a. group B antigens contain sialic acid
    b. group A antigens contain sialic acid
    c. group 0 antigens contain sialic acid
    d. each antigen of group B contains two residues of N-acetylgalactosamine
    e. each antigen of group B contains two residues of galactose

165. Glucidic residues that bind proteins by using a N- type bond usually bind to an asparagine residue embedded in this sequence (X=any amino acid; / = any of both posibilities)

    a. Asn-X-Asn/Gln
    b. Asn-X-Trp/Phe
    c. Asn-X-Tyr/Phe
    d. Asn-X-Asp/Glu
    e. Asn-X-Ser/Thr

166. Glucidic residues bound to collagen by an O- type bond are usually connected to two amino acid residues very characteristic of this protein, which are ...

    a. hydroxyproline and hydroxylysine
    b. acetyltyrosine and hidroxyproline
    c. hydroxytyrosine and hydroxyserine
    d. selenocysteine and 6-methylthreonine
    e. 2-OH-proline and 4-OH-alanine

Lipids

167. Fatty acids...

a. have a pK_a around 0.5, so they use to be anions at physiological pH
b. have a pK_a around 2.5, so they use to be anions at physiological pH
c. have a pK_a around 4.5, so they use to be anions at physiological pH
d. have a pK_a around 6.5, so they use to be anions at physiological pH
e. have a pK_a around 8.5, so they use to be anions at physiological pH

168. Myristic acid, also calle n-tetradecanoic acid, is named in abbreviated notation as 14:0. This indicates...

a. ...that it presents one unsaturated bond
b. ...that it is fully unsaturated
c. ...that it has no unsaturations
d. ...that its chemical formula is $CH_3(CH_2)_{10}COOH$
e. ...c and d are true

169. Oleic acid, also called cis-9-octadecenoic acid, is named in abbreviated notation as 18:1cΔ9. This indicates...

a. ...that it has one unsaturation of cis configuration
b. ...that has a minimum of 9 unsaturations, all them of cis configuration
c. ...that its chemical formula is $CH_3(CH_2)_7CH=CH(CH_2)_7COOH$
d. ...a and c are true
e. ...b and c are true

170. Below, some saturated fatty acids are listed, indicating in brackets the melting point in °C. Lignoceric acid (86,0); arachidic acid (76,5); lauric acid (44,2), stearic acid (69,6). Considering these data, it is true that...

a. ...arachidic acid has the largest number of carbons
b. ...lignoceric acid has more molecular weight than lauric acid
c. ...stearic acid presents more double bonds than lignoceric acid
d. ...if we order these molecules according to a crescent number of carbons, the order will be: lignoceric acid → arachidic acid → stearic acid → lauric acid
e. all the answers are TRUE

171. Abbreviated notation of all-cis-5,8,11,14-eicosatetraenoic acid (also called arachidonic acid) is writen as follows:

    a. 20:4cΔ5,8,11,14
    b. 22:4c
    c. 22:4cΔ14,11,8,5
    d. 22:4cΔ5,8,11,14
    e. 22:4c5,8,11,14

172. Which of the following sentences is FALSE?

    a. In most of the unsaturated fatty acids that are found in nature, the configuration of double bonds is trans
    b. Most of the fatty acids that are found in nature have an even number of carbon atoms
    c. Unsaturated fatty acids are those that have double bonds in its aliphatic chain
    d. Saturated fatty acids are those that do NOT have double bonds in its aliphatic chain
    e. Fatty acids are amphiphilic species

173. We name fats...

    a. ...to some molecules that are triesters of fatty acids and glycerol
    b. ...to the product of saponification of triglycerides
    c. ...to the whole fatty acids forming a micelle
    d. ...to the phosphate esters of fatty acids
    e. ...to the salts (generally sodic or potassic) of fatty acids

174. Fats...

    a. ...with high content in unsaturated fatty acids are liquid at room temperature
    b. ...with high content in saturated fatty acids are more watery than those that contain mainly unsaturated fatty acids
    c. ...that constitute olive oil have a low percentage (10-20%) of unsaturated fatty acids, such as oleic acid
    d. ...present in vegetables, such as fats of corn, are generally little watery and have to undergo hydrogenation to acquire liquid consistency
    e. All the options are TRUE

175. If fats are hydrolized with caustic soda (NaOH) or potash (KOH), we obtain...

a. ...micelles
b. ...soaps
c. ...phospholipids
d. ...more liquid fats
e. ...the complete saturation of their fatty acids

176. Soaps that come from saponification of fats have a problem in their domestic usage. Which is?

a. They get fully hydrogenated (saturated) Se hidrogenan completamente (se saturan) in contact with water, forming solid accumulations
b. In presence of hard waters (with high content in Ca^{2+} or Mg^{2+} cations) are transformed into fats
c. As they are sodium or potassium soaps (it occurs with the first ones in a higher Idegree), acidity notably increases in contact with water and can damage clothes
d. Are too soluble in water when compared with new generation synthetic soaps, such as sodium dodecyl sulfate (SDS)
e. In presence of hard waters (with high content in Ca^{2+} or Mg^{2+} cations), fatty acids precipitate, becoming useless to emulsify fats

177. We could define 'wax' as...

a. ...a short chain fatty acid esterified with a short chain alcohol
b. ...a short chain fatty acid esterified with a long chain alcohol
c. ...a long chain fatty acid esterified with a short chain alcohol
d. ...a long chain fatty acid esterified with a long chain alcohol
e. Neither is TRUE

178. Which of the following sentences is FALSE?

a. Hardness of waxes increases as the length and saturation level of fatty acids and alcohols forming them increase
b. Some marine microorganisms use waxes as energy source
c. Ester group (-COO-) confers certain hydrophilic degree to a molecule of wax
d. a wax is the product of the esterification of two long-chain fatty acids
e. Unsaturations introduced into hydrocarbon chains increase their fluidity

179. Which of the following phospholipids are most abundant in nature?

a. D-sphingophospholipids
b. L-glicerophospholipids
c. L-glycosphingolipids
d. D-glycoglycerolipids
e. L-glycoglycerolipids

180. Which of the following lists does contain only names of glycerophospholipids?

a. phosphatidic acid, phosphatidylcholine, phosphatidylinositol
b. phosphatidylethanolamine, sphingomyelin, ceramide
c. phosphatidylcholine, phosphatidylserine, cholesterol
d. phosphoric acid, phosphatidylcholine, phosphatidic acid
e. monogalactose diglyceride, phosphoserine, phosphatidylinositol

181. Which of the following molecules are glycerophospholipids?

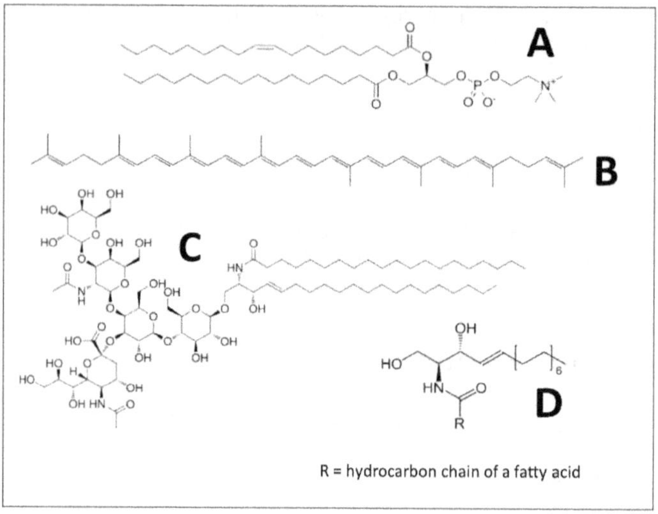

a. A
b. A and B
c. B
d. C and D
e. A and D

R = hydrocarbon chain of a fatty acid

182. The following table specifies the weight % of a series of membrane lipids in several types of cellular membranes.

According to data in the table, which of the following sentences is FALSE?

Lipid	In erythrocyte	In myelin	In cardiac cell mitochondria	In *E.coli*
Phosphatidic acid	1,5	0,5	0	0
Phosphatidylcholine	19	10	39	0
Phosphatidylethanolamine	18	20	27	65
Phosphatidylglycerol	0	0	0	18
Phosphatidylinositol	1	1	7	0
Phosphatidylserine	8	8	0,5	0
Sphingomyelin	17,5	8,5	0	0
Glycolipids	10	26	0	0
Cholesterol	25	26	3	0
Other	0	0	23,5	17

Data adapted from "Biochemistry of Mathews et al." (3ʳᵈ edition)

    a. in the studied examples about membranes of procaryotic cells, cholesterol is much more abundant than in the examples of membranes of eukaryotic cells
    b. glycerophospholipids constitute at least 50% of the composition of all the membranes analyzed
    c. in plasma membranes of eukaryotic cells (specifically in erythrocytes and myelin) cholesterol constitutes at least the 25 % of the whole lipids in the membrane
    d. sphingomyelin is not specially abundant in myelin, when compared to other eukaryotic tissues
    e. lipids derived from sphingosine esterification are absent in prokaryotes, in the cases analyzed

183. Which of the following molecules are sphingolipids?

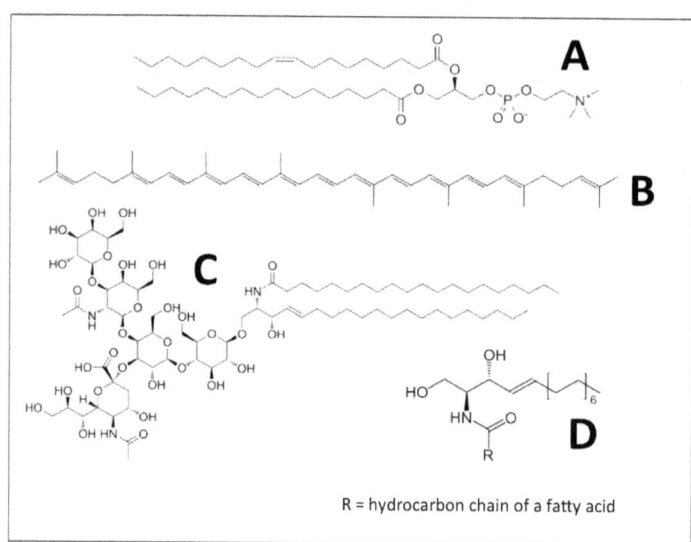

R = hydrocarbon chain of a fatty acid

a. A
b. B
c. C and A
d. D and C
e. A and D

184. Which of the following molecules is a glycosphingolipid?

R = hydrocarbon chain of a fatty acid

a. A
b. B
c. C
d. D
e. Neither

185. Which of the following molecules is a wax?

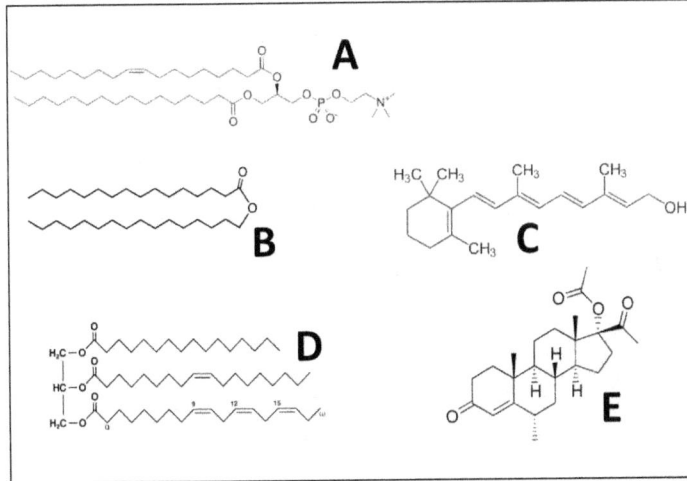

a. A
b. B
c. C
d. D
e. E

186. Which of the following molecules is a terpene?

a. A
b. B
c. C
d. D
e. E

187. Which of the following molecules is an steroid?

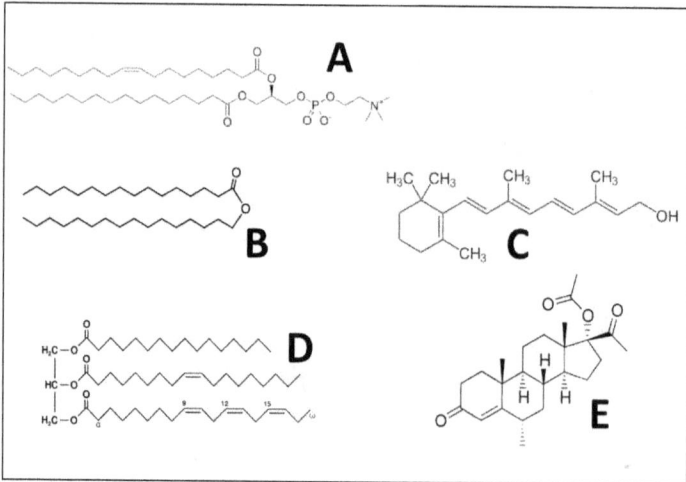

a. A
b. B
c. C
d. D
e. E

188. Which of the following molecules is a fat?

a. A
b. B
c. C
d. D
e. E

189. Which of the following molecules is a phospholipid?

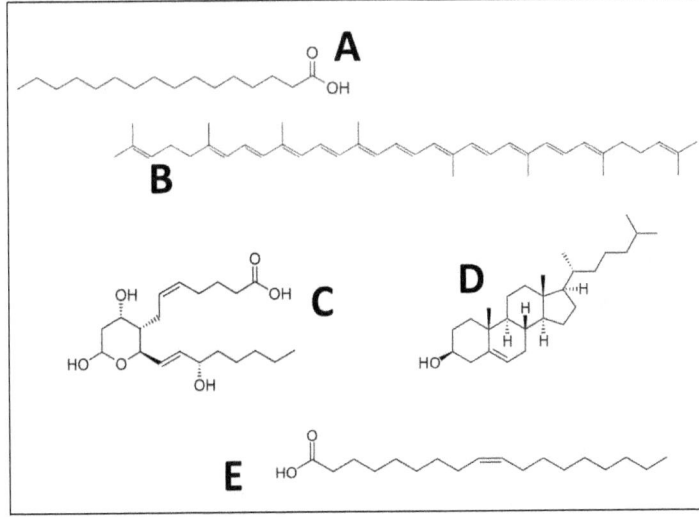

a. A
b. B
c. C
d. D
e. E

190. Which of the following molecules is an eicosanoid?

a. A
b. B
c. C
d. D
e. E

191. Which of the following molecules is a saturated fatty acid?

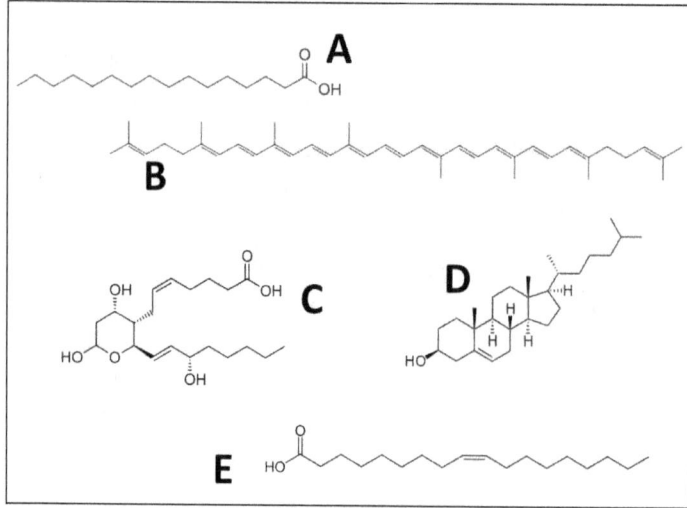

a. A
b. B
c. C
d. D
e. E

192. Which of the following molecules is cholesterol?

a. A
b. B
c. C
d. D
e. E

193. Which of the following molecules is an unsaturated fatty acids?

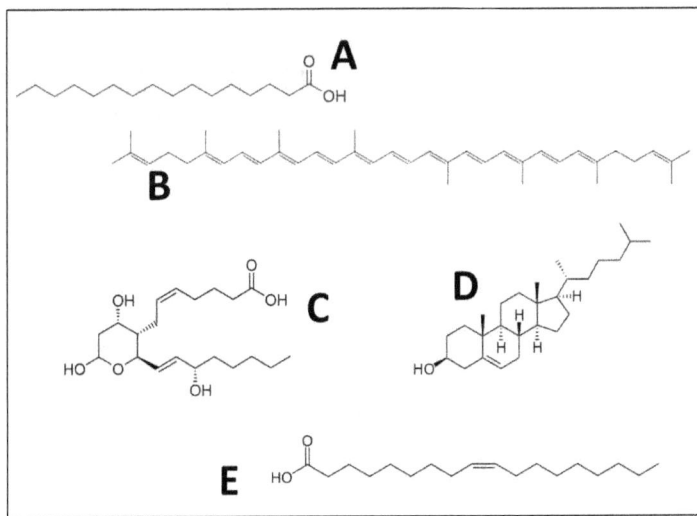

a. A
b. B
c. C
d. D
e. E

194. Which of the following molecules is a caroteneid pigment?

a. A
b. B
c. C
d. D
e. E

195. Glycerophospholipids...
A. ...are the most abundant phospholipids in nature
B. ...present in nature are mainly derived from the L enantiomer of glycerol-3-phosphate
C. ...have been found in bacteria, fungi, protists, plants and animals

a. All the sentences are TRUE
b. A and B are TRUE, C is FALSE
c. A is TRUE, B and C are FALSE
d. B is TRUE, A and C are FALSE
e. B and C are TRUE, A is FALSE

196. Glycerophospholipids derive from glycerol-3-phosphate, which of the following molecules is it?

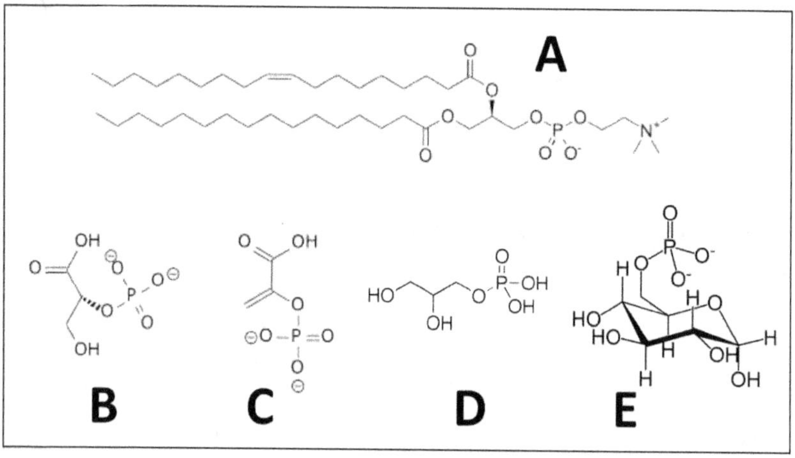

a. A
b. B
c. C
d. D
e. E

197. Which of the following fatty acids has the highest fusion temperature?
   A. 18:0
   B. 18:1cΔ9
   C. 18:1cΔ16
   D. 18:2cΔ9,16
   E. 18:3cΔ3,9,16

   a. A
   b. B
   c. C
   d. D
   e. E

198. Which of the following fatty acids has the highest fusion temperature?
   A. 22:1cΔ9
   B. 22:2tΔ9,16
   C. 22:2cΔ9,16
   D. 22:3cΔ3,9,16
   E. 22:3tΔ3,9,16

   a. A
   b. B
   c. C
   d. D
   e. E

199. Which of the following chemical groups is present in menthol?
   A. glycerol
   B. long chain alcohol
   C. phosphate group
   D. isoprene
   E. choline

   a. A and C
   b. A
   c. C and D
   d. D
   e. B

200. Which of the following chemical groups are present in waxes?
A. glycerol
B. long chain alcohol
C. phoshate group
D. monosaccharide
E. choline

a. A and B
b. B and C
c. C and E
d. B and C
e. B

201. Which of the following chemical groups is present in phosphatidylcholine?
A. glycerol
B. long-chain alcohol
C. phosphate group
D. isoprene
E. choline

a. A, B and C
b. A, B and D
c. A, B and E
d. A, C and E
e. A and C

202. Which of the following chemical structures is the linoleic acid?

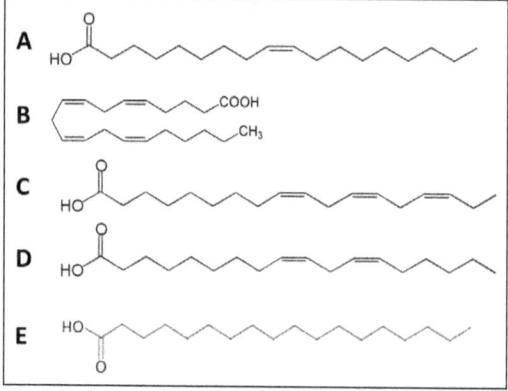

a. A
b. B
c. C
d. D
e. E

203. Which of the following chemical structures is the oleic acid?

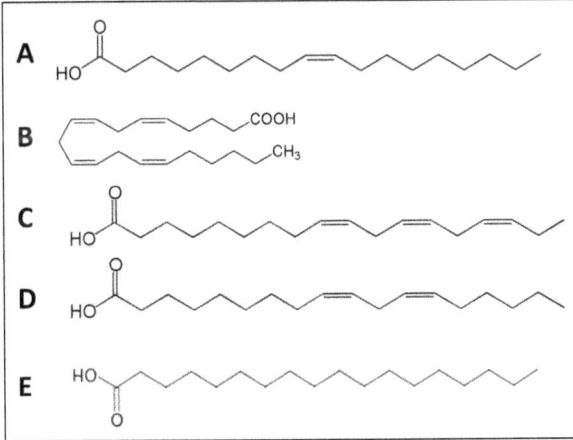

a. A
b. B
c. C
d. D
e. E

204. Which of the following structures is the stearic acid?

a. A
b. B
c. C
d. D
e. E

205. Which of the following structures is the α-linolenic acid?

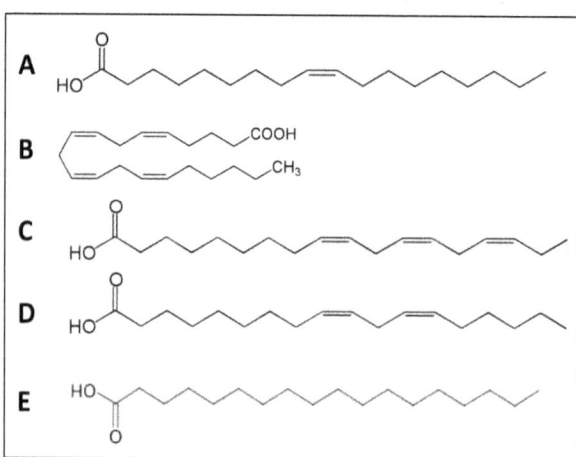

a. A
b. B
c. C
d. D
e. E

206. Which of the following structures is the arachidonic acid?

a. A
b. B
c. C
d. D
e. E

Biological membranes and transport

207. Fluid mosaic model, on biological membranes, was proposed in 1972 by...

a. S.J. Singer and G.L. Nicholson
b. S. Miller and J. Oró
c. P. Mitchell
d. J. Watson and F. Crick
e. F. Burlington and M. Perutz

208. In the book of W.M.Becker et al. ('The world of the cell', 2000) there is a curious study. Researchers fusion a mouse cell, in which membrane there are proteins labelled with red fluorescein, with a human cell in which membrane there are proteins labelled with green fluorescein. Which of the following results seems to be the one obtained?

a. A few minutes after membrane fusion, the distribution of red and green labelling is homogeneous and both markers are completely mixed.
b. Even hours after membrane fusion, red proteins remain located in a fixed zone in the membrane, whereas green ones freely diffuse.
c. Even hours after membrane fusion, green proteins remain located in a fixed zone in the membrane, whereas red ones freely diffuse.
d. Even hours after membrane fusion, red proteins remain located in a fixed zone in the membrane, and also green ones remain confined in a different location.
e. Some hours after cell fusion, all proteins expressed at the membrane level maintain a red fluorescence, thus indicating that mouse protein content prevails over human.

209. We perform the following experiment on a lipid bilayer composed by a 100% of dipalmitoylphosphatidylcholine. From an starting temperature of 0°C, we increase it progresively and measure by calorimetry the amount of heat absorved by the membrane (J/°C). Heat absortion presents a very sharp peak that starts at 35°C, achives its maximum at 40°C and returns to basal value at 45°C. What do you expect to occur in an analogous experiment if we add a 20% of cholesterol to the same membrane?

a. Heat absortion peak is almost equal in shape but it is displaced towards lower temperatures.
b. Heat absortion peak is almost equal in shape but it is displaced towards higher temperatures.
c. Heat absortion peak is much wider and softer. It affects a range of 30°C and the maximum value of heat is much lower than in the previous case. However, the temperature at which we fin the maximum value does not change.
d. Heat absortion peak is much wider and softer. It affects a range of 30°C and the maximum value of heat is much lower than in the previous case. Moreover, the temperature at which we fin the maximum value decreases.
e. Heat absortion peak is much wider and softer. It affects a range of 30°C and the maximum value of heat is much lower than in the previous case. Moreover, the temperature at which we fin the maximum value increases.

210. Gel-liquid transition temperature in a synthetic lipid bilayer give us an idea about its fluidity. A lipid bilayer of dipalmitoylphosphatidylcholine has a transition temperature of ~40°C. What would happen to this temperature if the same bilayer is completely built with a derivative of this phospholipid containing an unsaturation at the level of carbon 9 in each one of the hydrocarbon chains?

a. Temperature will not change, since it only depends on the number of carbons in the chain.
b. Temperature will slightly increase (around 5-10°C)
c. Temperature will notably increase (around 70-80°C)
d. Temperature will slightly decrease (around 5-10°C)
e. Temperature will notably decrease (around 70-80°C)

211. In reindeers, it has been observed that the cells that are next to the legs end have plasma membranes richer in unsaturated fatty acids than those that are next to the body. Which adaptative advantage do you think that this confers to reindeers?

a. None, since the unsaturation level of membrane phospholipds does not affect to gel-liquid transition temperature of the membrane.
b. It makes gel-liquid transition temperature to be much lower for the cells that we find far from the body than for those that are near the body, thus avoiding freezing of the distant ones.
c. It makes gel-liquid transition temperature to be much higher for the cells that we find far from the body than for those that are near the body, thus avoiding freezing of the distant ones.
d. It favours freezing of the cells at the end of the leg, triggering apoptotic processes and increasing cell renewal rate.
e. It allows the insertion of Ca^{2+} channels in plasma membrane, thus allowing a more intense drying of these cells and reducing its freezing risk.

212. Which of the following assertions is FALSE?

a. Human body cells, and the microorganisms hosted in the body, generally have in their plasma membranes a composition that allows transition temperature to be lower than body temperature.
b. Some even-toed ungulates (artiodactyla) like the reindeers, that live in cold places, it has been observed that the cells located far away from the body accumulate more unsaturations in the phospholipids of plasma membrane.
c. Adding cholesterol to a synthetic plasma membrane increases its transition temperature.
d. Movement of a free fatty acid between both faces of a plasma membrane is more favourable (when it comes to free energy) than the analogous movement made by a phospholipid.
e. The most common secondary structure in the protein segments that go across plasma membrane is α-helix.

213. Which of the following assertions, dealing with transport mechanisms across biological membranes, is FALSE?

a. facilitated diffusion systems that use only pores have a low dependency on temperature

b. facilitated diffusion systems that use only transporters have a notable dependency on temperature

c. transport rate in a mechanism of passive diffusion is directly proportional to the difference between the concentrations of the transported substance at both sides of the membrane

d. transport rate in a mechanism of active diffusion is directly proportional to the difference between the concentrations of the transported substance at both sides of the membrane

e. facilitated diffusion systems that use only pores have a low dependency on membrane fluidity

214. Usual values of concentration of Na$^+$ and K$^+$ in the extracellular environment of animals cells are, approximately...

a. $[Na^+]=140$ mM ; $[K^+]=5$ mM
b. $[Na^+]=1$ M ; $[K^+]=5$ µM
c. $[Na^+]=5$ mM ; $[K^+]=140$ mM
d. $[Na^+]=140$ µM ; $[K^+]=5$ µM
e. $[Na^+]=5$ µM ; $[K^+]=140$ µM

215. Usual values of concentration of Na$^+$ and K$^+$ in the cytosol of animals cells are, approximately...

a. $[Na^+]=100$ mM ; $[K^+]=10$ mM
b. $[Na^+]=10$ mM ; $[K^+]=10$ µM
c. $[Na^+]=10$ mM ; $[K^+]=10$ mM
d. $[Na^+]=10$ µM ; $[K^+]=100$ µM
e. $[Na^+]=10$ mM ; $[K^+]=100$ mM

216. A lipid bilayer has a thickness of ~3nm. How many residues of an α-helix fit in a transmembrane segment if the main axis of this segment does not bend at all?

a. 20
b. 30
c. 40
d. 50
e. 60

217. Which of the following drugs binds to α-chain of Na/K pump of cardiac muscle cells to exert its therapeutic effect?

    a. ouabain
    b. digitoxin
    c. indometacin
    d. a and b are true
    e. b and c are true

218. Na/K pump...

    a. ...pumps outside the cell 1 Na^+ for each 2 K^+ that introduces into cells
    b. ...pumps outside the cell 2 Na^+ for each 2 K^+ that introduces into cells
    c. ...pumps outside the cell 3 Na^+ for each 2 K^+ that introduces into cells
    d. ...pumps outside the cell 1 Na^+ for each 3 K^+ that introduces into cells
    e. ...pumps outside the cell 2 Na^+ for each 3 K^+ that introduces into cells

219. Valinomycin...

    a. ...is a transporter of K^+ cations
    b. ...adopts a folded form in which many atoms of N and O get located at the inner part, thus being able to chelate cations
    c. ...adopts a folded structure in which the external face is very hydrophobe, thus being able to move across the inner part of lipid bilayer
    d. a and b are true; c is false
    e. a, b and c are true

220. It has been suggested that Na/K pump, to couple ATP hydrolysis and cation transport, could be oscillating mainly between two conformations: a conformation opened to cytosol (C), and other opened to extracellular space (E). Relative to this, which of the following assertions is TRUE?

    a. C conformation favours K^+ intake and Na^+ release.
    b. E→C transition is triggered by the binding of ATP and the release of inorganic phosphate.
    c. C→E transition is triggered by phosphorilation of α subunit and ADP release.
    d. E conformation favours K^+ release.
    e. a and c are true.

221. Working of Na/K pump can be inhibited by cardiotonic steroids like ouabain or digitoxin. These drugs...

a. ...bind the pump preferably in its conformation opened to cytosol.
b. ...trigger the increase of [K+] at intracellular level.
c. ...cause an increase of [Na+] at intracellular level, which triggers mechanisms to eliminate the excess of Na+, like the activation of the Na+/Ca2+ interchanging pump.
d. ...as indirectly activate Na+/Ca2+ interchanging pump, increase [Ca2+] into sarcoplasmic reticulum of muscle cells, thus enhancing muscle contraction. So, they are used as cardiac stimulating drugs.
e. c and d are right.

222. Imagine a simplified model for ion transport across the membrane of a cell, in which only a given type of monovalent cation is involved, for example, Na+. In this model of cell, membrane potential ($\Delta\psi$) can be calculated by the following expression (Nernst's equation), where R is ideal gas constant, T is absolute temperature and F is Faraday's constant.

a. $\Delta\psi = (RTF) \cdot (\ln([Na^+]_{exterior}/[Na^+]_{interior}))$
b. $\Delta\psi = (RT/F) \cdot (\ln([Na^+]_{exterior}/[Na^+]_{interior}))$
c. $\Delta\psi = (RT/F) \cdot ([Na^+]_{exterior}/[Na^+]_{interior})$
d. $\Delta\psi = (RT/F) \cdot ([Na^+]_{interior}/[Na^+]_{exterior})$
e. $\Delta\psi = (RT/F) \cdot (\ln([Na^+]_{interior}/[Na^+]_{exterior}))$

223. For monovalent cations, Nernst's equation to compute electric potential of a biological membrane would have the following form, considering that we want the units of this potential ($\Delta\psi$) to be milivolts (mV).

a. $\Delta\psi = 59 \cdot \log_{10} ([cation]_{exterior}/[cation]_{interior})$
b. $\Delta\psi = 59 \cdot 10^{-3} \cdot \log_{10} ([cation]_{exterior}/[cation]_{interior})$
c. $\Delta\psi = -59 \cdot \log_{10} ([cation]_{exterior}/[cation]_{interior})$
d. $\Delta\psi = -59 \cdot 10^{-3} \cdot \log_{10} ([cation]_{exterior}/[cation]_{interior})$
e. $\Delta\psi = 59 \cdot \log_{10} ([cation]_{interior}/[cation]_{exterior})$

224. For monovalent anions, Nernst's equation to compute electric potential of a biological membrane would have the following form, considering that we want the units of this potential ($\Delta\psi$) to be milivolts (mV).

a. $\Delta\psi = 59 \cdot \log_{10} ([anion]_{exterior}/[anion]_{interior})$
b. $\Delta\psi = 59 \cdot 10^{-3} \cdot \log_{10} ([anion]_{exterior}/[anion]_{interior})$
c. $\Delta\psi = -59 \cdot \log_{10} ([anion]_{exterior}/[anion]_{interior})$
d. $\Delta\psi = -59 \cdot 10^{-3} \cdot \log_{10} ([anion]_{exterior}/[anion]_{interior})$
e. $\Delta\psi = 59 \cdot 10^{-6} \cdot \log_{10} ([anion]_{interior}/[anion]_{exterior})$

225. In squid neuron axon...

a. permeability is higher for Na^+ than for K^+
b. resting membrane potential is near -60mV
c. membrane potential can be computed through Goldman's equation, that requires we to know the permeability for each one of the ions present in the process
d. a and b are true
e. a, b and c are true

226. The treshold for the opening of sodium channels in the squid axon membrane is about -40mV. When this potential is reached, the most relevant observed effect is...

a. a massive entry of K^+ into the cell
b. a massive release of Na^+ from the cell
c. a massive entry of Na^+ into the cell
d. a massive release of K^+ from the cell
e. a massive entry of Ca^{2+} into the cell

227. Order the following events, corresponding to an excitability cycle in a neuron's membrane. The order must indicate their succession in time:
A. Sodium channels are closed and the K^+ release continues through specific voltage-dependent channels. This brings membrane potential to -70mV.
B. Membrane potential is about -60mV, similar to the membrane potential corresponding exclusively to K^+ action
C. Na^+ channels remain closed during a short period, this time they are resistant to opening (refractory period).
D. A massive entry of sodium, that brings membrane potential to +40mV, near to +55mV similar to the membrane potential corresponding exclusively to Na^+ action
E. Membrane potential rises to -40mV and voltage-dependent Na^+ channels are opened

a. B → D → E → A → C
b. E → B → D → C → A
c. B → E → A → D → C
d. B → C → E → D → A
e. B → E → D → A → C

228. Tetrodotoxin...

a. Binds specifically Na⁺ channels of axonal membrane and inhibits cationic flux.
b. Blocks specifically K⁺ channels of axonal membrane and inhibits cationic flux.
c. Triggers the opening of voltage-dependent Na⁺ channels, thus improving membrane permeability for these cations without needing previous voltage changes.
d. Triggers the opening of voltage-dependent K⁺ channels, thus improving membrane permeability for these cations without needing previous voltage changes .
e. None of the previous.

229. Saxitoxin...

a. Binds specifically Na⁺ channels of axonal membrane and inhibits cationic flux.
b. Blocks specifically K⁺ channels of axonal membrane and inhibits cationic flux.
c. Triggers the opening of voltage-dependent Na⁺ channels, thus improving membrane permeability for these cations without needing previous voltage changes.
d. Triggers the opening of voltage-dependent K⁺ channels, thus improving membrane permeability for these cations without needing previous voltage changes.
e. None of the previous.

230. Which of the following assertions, referring to veratridine, is true or false?
   A. Inhibits opening of Na⁺ channels
   B. Inhibits opening of K⁺ channels
   C. Stabilizes, through direct binding, the 'open' conformation of Na⁺ channels
   D. Is found in the seeds of a plant called *Schoenocaulon officinale*
   E. It's found in some organs of bubble-eye fishes, very appreciated in japanese culture

a. C and D are true, the rest are false
b. Only E is true
c. Only C and E are true
d. A, C and E are false, the rest are true
e. B, C and E are false, the rest are true

231. Tetrodotoxin...

a. ...can be found in the venom of vipers and other reptiles of dry environments
b. ...is made by cephalopods as a content of the ink and is used as a defense mechanism against predators
c. ...can be found in some organs of eye-bubbled fish
d. ...is present in some microscopic algae responsible for what we call 'red tide' (dinoflagellates) and can be incorporated to seafood that is nourished by these algae
e. ...can be found in a parasite of fishes called *Anisakis*

232. Saxitoxin...

a. ...can be found in the venom of vipers and other reptiles of dry environments
b. ...is made by cephalopods as a content of the ink and is used as a defense mechanism against predators
c. ...can be found in some organs of eye-bubbled fish
d. ...is present in some microscopic algae responsible for what we call 'red tide' (dinoflagellates) and can be incorporated to seafood that is nourished by these algae
e. ...can be found in a parasite of fishes called *Anisakis*

233. We have three lipid bilayers of rat erythrocytes. For each one of them, we measure the molar relationship between cholesterol (C) and phospholipids (PL), and indicate the value of the ratio in the following table.

	C:PL
Membrane X	0,2:1
Membrane Y	0,7:1
Membrane Z	1:1

Microscopic observation of the three membranes offers us the following data, some of which could be false.

A. Membrane X is narrower than membrane Y
B. In membrane Z we will find narrow islets formed basically by a cholesterol bilayer, and wider islets formed by a phospholipid bilayer with some content of inserted cholesterol
C. Membrane X is wider than Y
D. In membrane Y we will find narrow islets formed basically by a cholesterol bilayer, and wider islets formed by a phospholipid bilayer with some content of inserted cholesterol

a. Only A is true
b. Only C is true
c. Only A and B are true
d. Only A, B and D are true
e. Only B, C and D are true

234. A semipermeable membrane sepparates two compartments A and B. In these compartments there is a given solute at different concentrations (C_A and C_B). Variation of Gibbs free energy (ΔG) associated to the transport of 1 mol of solute through the membrane from A to B is given by the following equation:

a. $\Delta G = \ln(C_A/C_B)$
b. $\Delta G = RT\ln(C_A/C_B)$
c. $\Delta G = \ln(C_B/C_A)$
d. $\Delta G = RT\ln(C_B/C_A)$
e. $\Delta G = -T\ln(C_B/C_A)/R$

235. Net transport rate (J) of a given substance through a membrane by passive diffusion can be expressed in moles per squared centimetre per second, and is calculated by the following equation (where C_2 and C_1 are the concentrations at both sides of the membrane, I is the width of the membrane, D_1 is the diffusion coefficient for the substance and k is the partition coefficient between the lipid of the membrane and water, for this substance).

a. $J = kID_1(C_2-C_1)$
b. $J = (kD_1(C_2-C_1)/I)$
c. $J = (k(C_2-C_1)/(I\ D_1))$
d. $J = (D_1(C_2-C_1)/Ik)$
e. $J = I(kC_2-C_1D_1)$

236. Net transport rate (J) of a given substance through a membrane by passive diffusion can be expressed in moles per squared centimetre per second, and is calculated by the following equation (where C_2 and C_1 are the concentrations at both sides of the membrane, and P is the 'permeability coefficient' $P=kD_1/I$, where I is the width of the membrane, D_1 is the diffusion coefficient for the substance and k is the partition coefficient between the lipid of the membrane and water, for this substance).

a. $J = P(C_2-C_1)$
b. $J = (C_2-C_1)/P$
c. $J = -P(C_2-C_1)$
d. $J = -(C_2-C_1)/P$
e. $J = -(C_1-C_2)/P$

237. The ability, for a given substance, to diffuse across a lipid bilayer can be expressed by its 'permeability coefficient', that depends both on the substance and the membrane. Which of the following substances does present a higher permeability coefficient in a synthetic lipid bilayer of phosphatidylserine?

a. K^+
b. Na^+
c. Cl^-
d. Glucose
e. Water

238. Gramicidin A...

a. ...acts as an specific pore for cation transport across membranes
b. ...enhances the pass of K^+ cations and, to a lower extent, of the Na^+ cations
c. ...acts as a dimer
d. a and b are true; c is false
e. a, b and c are true

239. In a facilitated diffusion process of a substance A through a membrane, if we represent transport rate in y-axis and in the x-axis we represent the difference among the concentration of substance A at both sides of the membrane, which will be the form of the resulting graph?

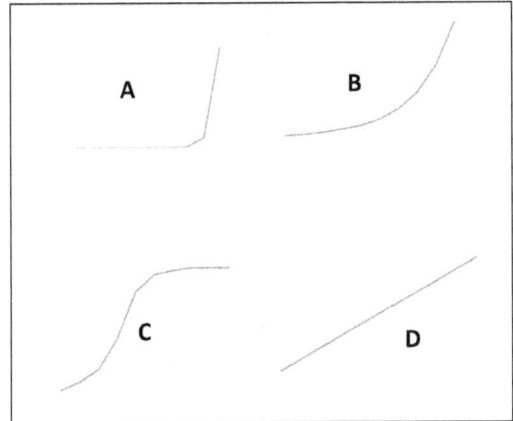

a. A
b. B
c. C
d. D
e. A or B depending on the initial concentration of membrane transporters

240. In a simple diffusion process of a substance A through a membrane, if we represent transport rate in y-axis and in the x-axis we represent the difference among the concentration of substance A at both sides of the membrane, which will be the form of the resulting graph?

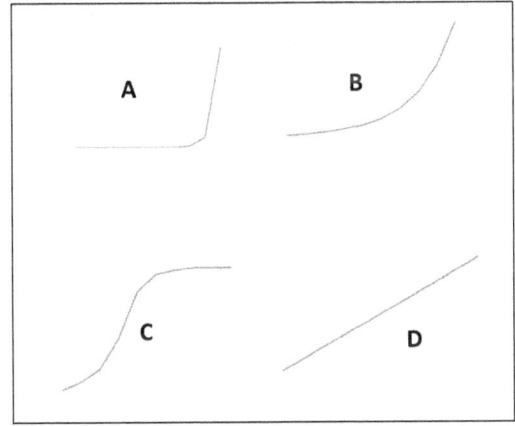

a. A
b. B
c. C
d. D
e. A or B depending on the initial concentration of membrane transporters

Proteins: amino acids and peptides

241. Which of the following amino acids has a positive charge in its lateral chain at physiological pH?

a. glycine
b. aspartic acid
c. serine
d. tyrosine
e. lysine

242. What is glutathione?

a. it is a tripeptide of glutamate, cysteine and glycine that allows the regulation of redox potential in most of the cells
b. it is a dipeptide formed by aspartic acid and glycine. It is used as artificial sweetener
c. it is a small protein (33 amino acids) that antagonizes hormonal effects of insulin, thus regulating blood sugar levels
d. it is the monovalent anion of glutamic acid, that is only found in solution at neutral pH, since it is dianionic at a lower pH
e. it is a measure of the capacity of a given solution of amino acids as pH buffering agent

243. Which of the following amino acids does NOT present a cyclic group in its lateral chain?

a. phenylalanine
b. glutamine
c. tyrosine
d. tryptophan
e. histidine

244. Imagine that you have a solution (at neutral pH) with concentrations 0,05 M for each one of the following amino acids. When pH rises from 7 to 12, which of them will be the first in losing a proton from its lateral chain?

a. phenylalanine
b. glutamine
c. tyrosine
d. tryptophan
e. histidine

245. X-ray crystallography can determine the approximated position of each one of the heavy atoms (C,N,O,S) of a protein, but it has no resolution enough to see the position of hydrogens. Thus, 3D structures determined by X-ray offer us a view of the protein without hydrogens. By considering the pH of solution, we can know if a lateral chain of an amino acid will be protonated or not. For most amino acids, in a pH range between 6 and 8, this is an easy task, since the protonation state of lateral chains does not vary in this range. There is an exception to this behaviour. It's the amino acid...

a. phenylalanine
b. glutamine
c. tyrosine
d. tryptophan
e. histidine

246. Phenylketonuria ia a genetic disease characterized by the disability of the patient to transform phenylalanine into tyrosine. It's usually due to the lack of the enzyme phenylalanine hydrolase or the enzyme tetrahydrobiopterin reductase. What is observed in patients of such disease?

a. they are fair, since tyrosine is a precursor in melanin synthesis
b. they show an increase of phenylketonuria in urine
c. their diet needs to be complemented by tyrosine
d. a, b and c are right
e. only b and c are right

247. Which of the following amino acids is represented by the letter W?

a. tryptophan
b. tyrosine
c. phenylalanine
d. valine
e. threonine

248. Proteins can be N-glycosylated in some residues. Which is the most common form?

    a. A residue of N-acetylglucosamina bound to the amide nitrogen of any peptide bond
    b. A residue of N-acetylglucosamina bound to the amine nitrogen of a lysine
    c. A residue of N-acetylglucosamina bound to the amide nitrogen of a glutamine
    d. A residue of N-acetylglucosamina bound to the amide nitrogen of an asparagine
    e. A residue of N-acetylglucosamina bound to the amide nitrogen of an arginin

249. The most abundant amino acids in proteins are...

    a. L-α-amino acids
    b. D-α-amino acids
    c. L-β-amino acids
    d. D-β-amino acids
    e. Answers b anc d are rigth

250. Which of the following amino acids is represented by the letter Q?

    a. isoleucine
    b. tyrosine
    c. phenylalanine
    d. arginine
    e. glutamine

251. Which of the following amino acids is represented by the letter R?

    a. aspartic acid
    b. threonine
    c. asparagine
    d. arginine
    e. glutamine

252. The figure shows acid base equilibrium for alanine and the pK_a values associated to each reaction. If the concentration of A is 0,8 M and the concentration of B is 0.4 M, what is the pH of the solution?

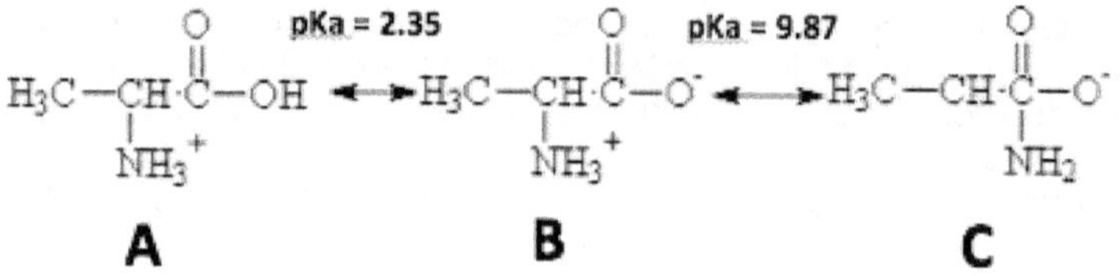

$pKa = 2.35$ $pKa = 9.87$

$$H_3C—CH·\overset{O}{\overset{\|}{C}}—OH \longleftrightarrow H_3C—CH·\overset{O}{\overset{\|}{C}}—O^- \longleftrightarrow H_3C—CH·\overset{O}{\overset{\|}{C}}—O^-$$

    $\overset{|}{N}H_3^+$ $\overset{|}{N}H_3^+$ $\overset{|}{N}H_2$

A   **B**   **C**

a. 1.66
b. 2.05
c. 2.65
d. 3.04
e. 6.11

253. Which of the following amino acids has a positive charge in its lateral chain at physiological pH?

a. phenylalanine
b. glutamine
c. valine
d. tyrosine
e. arginine

254. Proteins can undergo O-glycosylation in some residues, which is the most common form?

a. A residue of N-acetylgalactosamine bound to a residue of valine or histidine
b. A residue of N-acetylgalactosamine bound to a residue of tryptophan or tyrosine
c. A residue of N-acetylgalactosamine bound to a residue of alanine or glutamine
d. A residue of N-acetylgalactosamine bound to a residue of glycine or alanine
e. A residue of N-acetylgalactosamine bound to a residue of serine or threonine

255. Which of the following amino acids has a negative charge in its lateral chain at physiological pH?

    a. glutamine
    b. glutamic acid
    c. lysine
    d. a and b are true
    e. b and c are true

256. X-ray crystallography can determine the approximated position of each one of the heavy atoms (C,N,O,S) of a protein, but it has no resolution enough to see the position of hydrogens. Thus, 3D structures determined by X-ray offer us a view of the protein without hydrogens. By considering the pH of solution, we can know if a lateral chain of an amino acid will be protonated or not. For most amino acids, in a pH range between 6 and 8, this is an easy task, since the protonation state of lateral chains does not vary in this range. There is an exception to this behaviour. It's the amino acid...

    a. phenylalanine
    b. glutamine
    c. aspartic acid
    d. asparagine
    e. histidine

257. Following sentences refer to the investigations on the origin of L vs D preference in amino acid chirality. Indicate which of the assertions is FALSE.

    a. In the α-methyl-amino acids found in Murchison meteorite (Australia, 1969) a slight preference for L forms is detected.
    b. In Strecker reactions, amino acids are generated as a racemic mixture
    c. Polarized light from some stars seems that partially destroys D forms of amino acids
    d. An important problem is that the transformation of α-methyl-amino to α-amino acids in natural conditions has not been currently achieved
    e. The loss of L preference (racemization) in amino acids can be used as a measure of time in corpse dating methods

258. Following figure shows acid-base equilibrium for histidine, indicating pK$_a$ value for each reaction. Based on these data, which is the value of the isoelectric point (pI) of histidine?

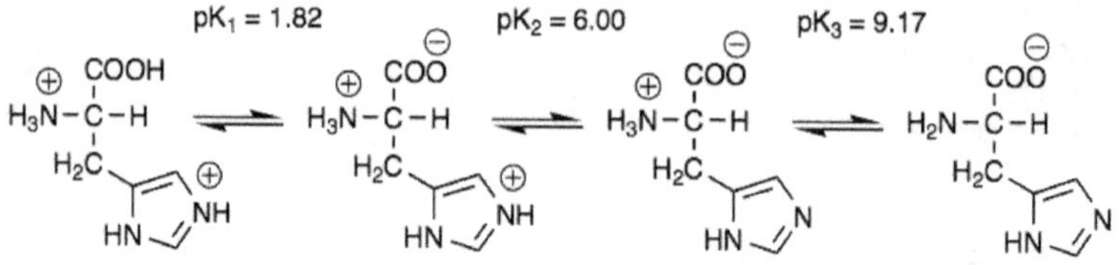

$$pK_1 = 1.82 \qquad pK_2 = 6.00 \qquad pK_3 = 9.17$$

a. 3.91
b. 5.50
c. 5.66
d. 7.59
e. 8.50

259. Which of the following amino acids is represented by the letter Y?

a. tryptophan
b. tyrosine
c. phenylalanine
d. valine
e. threonine

260. Molecular basis for different blood types in the ABO system is based on the nature of some oligosaccharides bound to erythrocyte surface proteins. Which of the following assertions concerning oligosaccharides is TRUE?

a. they are O-glycosylations in which the following sugars are involved: fucose, galactose, N-acetylgalactosamine and sialic acid
b. they are O-glycosylations in which the following sugars are involved: glucose and galactose
c. they are N-glycosylations in which the following sugars are involved: N-acetylgalactosamine and sialic acid
d. they are N-glycosylations in which the following sugars are involved: N-acetylgalactosamine, N-acetylglucosamine, glucose and sialic acid
e. they are O-glycosylations in which the following sugars are involved: fucose, fructose and sialic acid

261. Some amino acids in proteins can be phosphorylated, which are they?

a. aspartic acid, serine, leucine
b. glycine, phenylalanine, threonine
c. valine, glutamic acid, aspartic acid
d. alanine, lysine, glutamine
e. tyrosine, serine, threonine

262. Which of the following amino acids has the bulkiest lateral chain?
a. glycine
b. leucine
c. tryptophan
d. valine
e. serine

263. Isoelectric point of an amino acid is...

a. the pH at which amino acid charge is 0
b. the pK_a at whichen el que la carga del amino acid es 0
c. the pK_a added to the logarithm of the ratio between the concentrations of the protonated and unprotonated form of an amino acid
d. the pK_a added to the logarithm of the ratio between the concentrations of the unprotonated and protonated form of an amino acid
e. the average of all the pK_a values associated to this amino acid

264. Which of the following amino acids can form disulphide bridges in proteins?

a. cysteine
b. threonine
c. serine
d. tyrosine
e. lysine

265. N-linked oligosaccharides bind to proteins mainly through an asparagine thet is found in the following amino acid sequence ("X" indicates any amino acid, "/" indicates alternance between two or more amino acids)...

a. Asn-X-X-X-Glu-Pro
b. Asn-X-Ser/Thr
c. Pro-Asn-X-His
d. Gly/Ala-X-Asn-Phe/Trp
e. Asn-X-Glu/Asp

266. Which of the following amino acids is represented by the letter T?

a. tryptophan
b. tyrosine
c. thymine
d. thiamine
e. threonine

267. Cation-π interactions...

a. can occur between a cation like sodium and an amino acid like glutamine
b. can occur between the lateral chain of a tyrosine and that of an alanine
c. can occur between a cation and the lateral chain of asparagine
d. can occur between lysine and phenylalanine
e. a and d are true

268. β-alanine is a precursor of Coenzyme A synthesis. An intermediate of this synthesis is used in cosmetics industry (creams, shampoos,...) as an skin growth enhancer. We are talking about...

a. pantothenic acid
b. ornithine
c. phenylalanine
d. glucagon
e. myosin

269. Which of these assertions is FALSE.

a. Dermorphin is a protein isolated from the skin of some frogs and has an anesthetic effect acting on opioid receptors in human central nervous system.
b. Dermorphin has an amino acid of the isomer form D, specifically the second one, that is a D-tyrosine.
c. Nisin is a food preservative of peptidic nature.
d. Aspartame is used as sweetener and is of peptidic nature.
e. Some snails use acathin-I, an small peptide that contains D-phenylalanine and enhances muscular contraction.

270. Which of the following amino acids is represented by the letter K?

a. lysine
b. cysteine
c. glutamic acid
d. arginine
e. tyrosine

271. Which of the following amino acids is represented by the letter E?

a. methionine
b. aspartic acid
c. glutamic acid
d. asparagine
e. phenylalanine

272. Molecular basis of the different blood types of the ABO system is based on the nature of some pentasaccharides bound to erythrocyte surface proteins. Which is the difference between A and B antigens?

a. a galactose present in A is absent in B
b. a galactose present in A is substituted by a glucose in B
c. a sialic acid present in A is changed by an N-acetylgalactosamine in B
d. an N-acetylgalactosamine present in A is substituted by a galactose in B
e. a fructose present in A is substituted by a glucose in B

273. Which of the following amino acids is represented by the letter D?

a. serine
b. aspartic acid
c. glutamic acid
d. histidine
e. valine

274. Which of the following amino acids has a negative charge in its lateral chain at physiological pH?

a. asparagine
b. aspartic acid
c. serine
d. a and b are right
e. b and c are right

275. Ornithine is an important derivative of natural amino acids, which of the following chemical structures does represent this molecule?

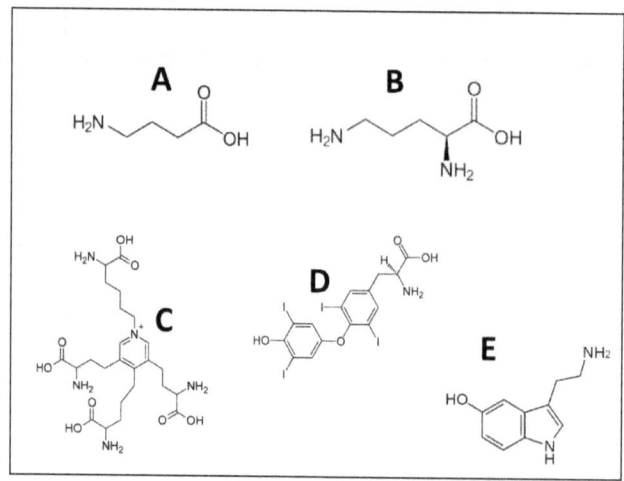

a. A
b. B
c. C
d. D
e. E

276. γ-aminobutyric acid (GABA) is an important derivative of natural amino acids, which of the following chemical structures does represent this molecule?

a. A
b. B
c. C
d. D
e. E

277. Serotonin is an important derivative of natural amino acids, which of the following chemical structures does represent this molecule?

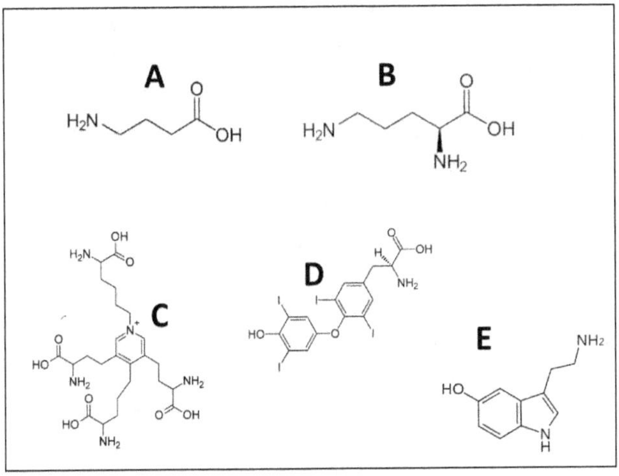

a. A
b. B
c. C
d. D
e. E

278. Desmosine is an important derivative of natural amino acids, which of the following chemical structures does represent this molecule?

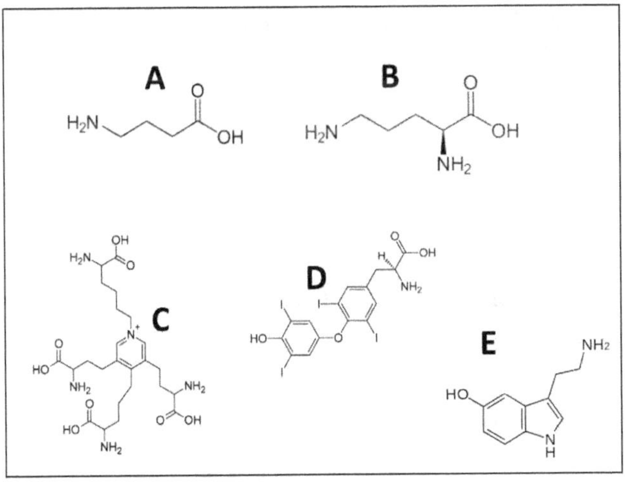

a. A
b. B
c. C
d. D
e. E

279. Thyroxine is an important derivative of natural amino acids, which of the following chemical structures does represent this molecule?

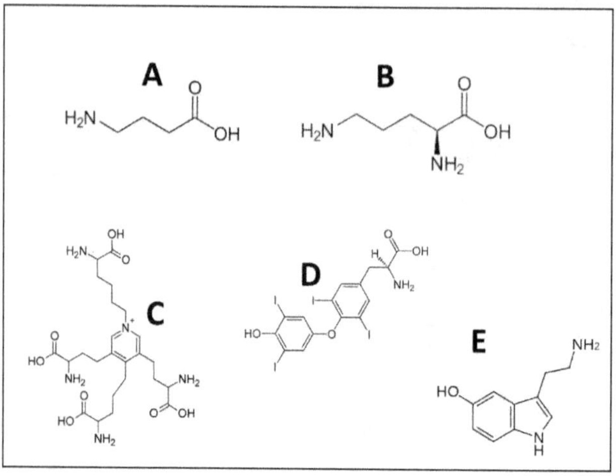

a. A
b. B
c. C
d. D
e. E

280. Melanocyte-stimulating hormone is a peptide of 13 amino acids that was firstly described by A.B. Lerner (Yale University). There are several forms and its role is to stimulate melanocyte proliferation in vertebrates. A common sequence is the following:

Ser-Tyr-Ser-Met-Glu-His-Phe-Arg-Trp-Gly-Lys-Pro

What is the proper way of writing it with the 1-letter code?

a. STSMGHFRWGLP
b. SYSMUHFRWGLP
c. SYSMEHFRWGKP
d. SYSMDHFRWGKP
e. SYSMEHFAWGKP

281. Which of the following amino acids is the most hydrophobic?

a. phenylalanine
b. glutamine
c. glutamic acid
d. aspartic acid
e. glycine

282. Gluthatione peroxidase contains some special residues, similar to cysteine, in which a sulphur atom has been substituted by another element, which is this element?

a. Nickel
b. Selenium
c. Silver
d. Boron
e. Oxygen

283. Which of the following amino acids is the smallest one?

a. phenylalanine
b. glutamine
c. glutamic acid
d. aspartic acid
e. glycine

Proteins: structure

284. In an α-helix...

a. helix turns in a levorotary way
b. phi angle in amino acids is maintained around -140°
c. N-terminal ends are specially rich in lysine or arginine
d. we find 3.6 amino acids for each helix turn
e. b and d are right

285. A collagen helix...

a. has 3.6 amino acids for each turn
b. has 5.4 amino acids for each turn
c. has 4.4 amino acids for each turn
d. is an structure formed by 3 chains. Each one of them is a levorotary helix
e. c and d are right

286. Ramachandran's plot...

a. is a graphical representation of phi and psi angles for each amino acid in a protein
b. is the diagram that relates polarity of amino acids to their propensity to be within β-sheet structures
c. is a 20 x 20 matrix containing interaction energy between all amino acids, representing such energy by a colour scale
d. is the graphical representation of Henderson-Hasselbalch equation for a given amino acid. X-axis indicates the pH of a pure 1 M solution of this amino acid, and Y-axis indicates the concentration of zwitterion species
e. was proposed by Cyrus Levinthal in 1969, and it tries to explain graphically Levinthal's paradox

287. Observe the following sequence and A, B, C, D and E stretches. Indicate which of the following assertions is FALSE.

B

(N-terminal) ...AKRLKNGWAVLFILIYKAWQRPACERGLQILENCASTEDFGTRYHC... (C-terminal)

A   C   D   E

a. B strectch holds a distribution of aromatic residues typical in an α helix
b. D stretch can form a β turn more probably than C stretch
c. in the whole sequence there are more charged residues than aromatic
d. A stretch can form an α helix with a high probability
e. the ends of E stretch could be bound by a disulfide bridge

288. In an α-helix ...

a. each oxygen of the carbonyl group of the main chain interacts through a H-bond with the proton of the amide group of the next residue in the helix
b. each oxygen of the carbonyl group of the main chain interacts through a H-bond with the proton of the amide group of the residue that is in the second place from it in the helix
c. each oxygen of the carbonyl group of the main chain interacts through a H-bond with the proton of the amide group of the residue that is in the third place from it in the helix
d. each oxygen of the carbonyl group of the main chain interacts through a H-bond with the proton of the amide group of the residue that is in the fourth place from it in the helix
e. each oxygen of the carbonyl group of the main chain interacts through a H-bond with the proton of the amide group of the residue that is in the fifth place from it in the helix

289. In an α-helix, each H-bond between the carbonyl and the amide group in different residues in main chain stabilizes this secondary structure. When it comes to geometry, this H-bond closes a loop of covalently attached atoms. How many atoms are there in the loop?

a. The number of atoms extremely varies depending on sequence
b. 13
c. 15
d. 17
e. 19

290. In a 3_{10} helix, each H-bond between the carbonyl and the amide group in different residues in main chain stabilizes this secondary structure. When it comes to geometry, this H-bond closes a loop of covalently attached atoms. How many atoms are there in the loop?

a. The number of atoms extremely varies depending on sequence
b. 3
c. 7
d. 10
e. 13

291. In a π helix (also called $4,4_{16}$ helix), each H-bond between the carbonyl and the amide group in different residues in main chain stabilizes this secondary structure. When it comes to geometry, this H-bond closes a loop of covalently attached atoms. How many atoms are there in the loop?

a. The number of atoms extremely varies depending on sequence
b. 4
c. 8
d. 12
e. 16

292. In folded β-sheet, all residues present a rotation in relation to the previous residue. Of how many degrees is this rotation?

a. 12°
b. 45°
c. 60°
d. 90°
e. 180°

293. Individual chains that form a collagen triple helix (a tropocollagen unit), are...

a. dextrorotary helices of ~3.9 residues per turn
b. levorotary helices of ~3.9 residues per turn
c. dextrorotary helices of ~3.6 residues per turn
d. levorotary helices of ~3.3 residues per turn
e. dextrorotary helices of ~3.3 residues per turn

294. Tropocollagen is the main unit constituting collagen fibers. A unit of tropocollagen consists in 3 helices coiled one with the other. It's curious that, in each one of these helices, each 3 residues we almost always find an amino acid called...

a. glycine
b. alanine
c. valine
d. tryptophan
e. asparagine

295. In collagen, it appears with a high frequency an amino acid derived from natural amino acids naturales, it is...

a. isovaline
b. selenocysteine
c. hydroxyproline
d. aspartame
e. pantothenic acid

296. In collagen...

a. hydroxylysine residues are anchoring points for polysaccharides
b. hydroxyproline residues confer mechanical stability
c. hydroxylysine residues are the most frequent covalent modifications present in this protein
d. a and b are right
e. b and c are right

297. Fibroin is a protein that confers a high mechanical resistance to silk and spider webs. Its structure is very rich in β-sheet regions, that are specially resistant. The sequence of these regions is characteristic since it contains, almost each 2 residues, the amino acid...

    a. phenylalanine
    b. glutamine
    c. glutamic acid
    d. aspartic acid
    e. glycine

298. α-keratins are proteins basically formed by α-helix structures. It's quite frequent to kfind that, every two α-helices, get coiled in a higher levorotary superstructure. This so specific superstructrure can be formed in α-keratins for the following reason...

    a. each α-helix has an slight levorotary coiling. So, the fitting of 2 of these structures is just due to a simple steric coupling.
    b. each 4 amino acids, α-keratins present an hydrophobe residue. Since α-helix has 3.6 amino acids for each turn, these hydrophobe residues remain almost aligned in the same face. Hydrophobe residues tend to be together and so helices are bound by these points. The small unfit between 4 (distance between hydrophobe residues) and 3.6 (amino acids needed to complete a turn around the helix) produces an slight levorotary coiling.
    c. α-keratins are rich in aromatic residues. This kind of residues appear on average each 8-10 residues. Stacking interactions between aromatic residues allow a pair of α-keratins to be perfectly bound by these points. Resulting structure is not very soluble and, for this reason, an slight levorotary helicity is generated.
    d. α-keratins are rich in aromatic residues. This kind of residues appear on average each 8-10 residues. Stacking interactions between aromatic residues allow a pair of α-keratins to be perfectly bound by these points. Since the distance of 8-10 residues does not match exactly with an integer number of helix turns (but it is equivalent to a range of 2.2-2.8 turns) aromatic residues are not located in the same face of the helix and, to reach the highest energetic stability, an slight levorotary helicity is generated.
    e. none of the previous explanations is right to explain the left rotation normally found in bound α-keratins.

299. In collagen fibers, for the fiber to be harder, the units of tropocollagen are interlinked by covalent bonds (formed by oxidation, aldol condensation and dehydration) between some specific amino acids, which are these amino acids?

a. lysines
b. glutamines
c. asparagines
d. arginines
e. histidines

300. Different turns (α, β, γ, δ) of peptide chain in globular proteins are named according to the number of peptide bonds that separate the first and last residue in the turn. In this way...

a. α turns are those in which first and last residue are separated by 2 bonds
b. β turns (the most abundant) are those in which first and last residue are separated by 3 bonds
c. δ turns are those in which first and last residue are separated by 2 bonds
d. a and b are right
e. b and c are right

301. Carbohydrate residues that bind proteins through N-type bonds, are linked to residues of ...

a. serine
b. threonine
c. methionine
d. asparagine
e. phenylalanine

302. Oligosaccharides that bind proteins through N-type bonds, use normally as the monosaccharides bound to asparagine...

a. glucose or N-acetylglucose
b. N-acetylglucosamine or N-acetylgalactosamine
c. mannose or trehalose
d. mannitol or sorbitol
e. N-acetylpyridine o N-methylglucosamine

303. Oligosaccharides bound to proteins through an O-type bond, usually form a bond between _____ and the hydroxyl group of _____ or _____.

a. N-acetylgalactosamine / threonine / serine
b. galactosamine / phenylalanine / tyrosine
c. N-methylglucosamine / phenylalanine / tyrosine
d. glucosamine / threonine / serine
e. N-methylglucosamine / threonine / serine

304. Sugar residues that bind proteins through an N-type bond usually bind to an asparagine residue embedded in the following sequence (X=any amino acid; / = one of both possibilities)

a. Asn-X-Asn/Gln
b. Asn-X-Trp/Phe
c. Asn-X-Tyr/Phe
d. Asn-X-Asp/Glu
e. Asn-X-Ser/Thr

305. Sugar residues that bind to collagen by an O-type bond usually bind to 2 modified amino acids typical of this protein, which are these residues?

a. hydroxyproline and hydroxylysine
b. acetyltyrosine and hydroxyproline
c. hydroxytyrosine and hydroxyserine
d. selenocysteine and 6-methylthreonine
e. 2-OH-proline and 4-OH-alanine

Proteins: function

306. Chaperones...

a. are proteins specialized in accelerating and driving protein folding process
b. are proteins that eliminate proline residues from α-helices
c. have mainly the role of stimulating thyrotropin secretion in pituitary gland
d. are small proteins (29 residues), among which we find examples like insulin, glucagon or corticotropin
e. are proteins secreted by macrophages to the extracellular environment, involved in dissolving the wall of some bacteria

307. Indicate which assertion is FALSE

a. α-keratins are proteins very abundant in hair, nails, wool or horns
b. α-keratins are composed by a high proportion of α-helices
c. α-keratins were the material on which William Astbury observed the repeats of patterns each 5,15-5,20 angstroms, that led him to the description of α-helices
d. α-keratins are highly soluble in water
e. α-keratins are specially rich in hydrophobe residues

308. Proteins...

a. have a tertiary structure that remains rigid to play their biological role
b. can have different binding sites for several ligands
c. have a unique binding site for each ligand
d. bind their ligands in an irreversible way, through covalent bonds
e. can undergo drastic conformational changes, in the order of nanometers

309. We call induced fit to ...

a. the loss of disulfide bridges between cysteines
b. the adjustments in the expression levels of a given protein
c. the adjustments in the expression levels of the active site of a given protein
d. the structural adaptation that a protein undergoes to better bind to its ligand
e. the spatial adjustment of solvent molecules around the active site of a protein

310. Which of the following assertions is FALSE?

a. if a molecule binds to an enzyme, that catalyzes its conversion into a new product, we call it substrate

b. if a molecule binds to an enzyme, that catalyzes its conversion into a new product by breaking/formation of covalent bonds, we call it substrate

c. if a molecule binds to a protein in a reversible way and is not covalently modified we call it ligand

d. O_2 is a ligand for hemoglobin

e. lactate is a ligand for lactate dehydrogenase

311. Which of the following assertions on myoglobin is right?

a. It was firstly described in the middle of 20th century

b. It was firstly purified in 1958, by John Kendrew

c. Its 3D structure was solved by X-ray in 1958, by Max Perutz

d. The discovery of its 3D structure deserved the Nobel Prize in Chemistry in 1962

e. Its 3D structure was described only 1 year after the one of hemoglobin

312. In myoglobin...

a. heme group is located in the cleft between helices E and F, although it also interacts with residues in other segments

b. heme group is located in the cleft between helices A and B, although it also interacts with residues in other segments

c. heme group is located in the cleft between helices A and F, although it also interacts with residues in other segments

d. heme group is located in the cleft between helices A and C, although it also interacts with residues in other segments

e. heme group is located in the cleft between helices B and F, although it also interacts with residues in other segments

313. Myoglobin...

a. has 351 amino acids and 8 α-helix segments
b. has 351 amino acids, 8 α-helix segments connected by turns, and presents a non-helicoidal small region
c. has 153 amino acids, 8 α-helix segments connected by turns, and presents a non-helicoidal small region from amino acid 100 to 107
d. has 153 amino acids, 8 α-helix segments connected by turns, and presents in a non-helicoidal way the two first N-terminal residues and the 5 last C-terminal residues
e. has 351 amino acids, 8 α-helix segments connected by turns, and presents a small region, of 14 amino acids, that forms an small β-sheet in the C-terminal zone

314. Which of the following assertions is FALSE?

a. If blood Fe^{2+} was not mainly bound to heme group of haemoglobin, it would cause the generation of oxygen reactive species (hydroxyl radicals, etc.)
b. Hemoglobin is constituted by 4 proteic subunits
c. Heme group has 4 nitrogens that form bonds to Fe^{2+} in the plane of porphyrin, leaving two coordination loci free to bind O_2
d. Electrophilic nature of nitrogens in heme group prevents oxidation from Fe^{2+} to Fe^{3+}
e. Iron present in heme group binds O_2 if it's in its reduced form (Fe^{2+}) and does not bind O_2 if it's in its oxidized form (Fe^{3+})

315. We call hemoproteins...

a. to the proteins present in blood
b. to the metalloproteins that have heme group as prosthetic group
c. to the proteins constituted by two subunits of identical sequence
d. to the proteins that share a high sequence identity (>50%, generally) with hemoglobin, for instance myoglobin, peroxidases and catalase
e. to the proteins that bind Fe^{2+} and O_2

316. Which of the following assertions regarding blood coagulation is FALSE?

a. The breaking of fibrinogen by the action of thrombin generates fibrin
b. The breaking of fibrinogen by the action of thrombin, besides fibrin, generates two small peptides called fibrinopeptides A and B
c. Striations of a fibrin fiber have an approximate separation of 23 nm
d. Activated XII factor activates XI factor
e. In damaged tissues, quininogen and kallikrein proteins activate XII factor, thus initiating the extrinsic pathway of blood coagulation

317. Which of the following lists does contain only hemoproteins...

a. hemoglobin, myoglobin, myosin and ferredoxin
b. peroxidase, leghemoglobin, cytochrome C and hemoglobin
c. hemoglobin, myosin, cytochrome C oxidase, lactate dehydrogenase
d. lactate dehydrogenase, pyruvate carboxylase, myoglobin and catalase
e. catalase, glucokinase, leghemoglobin, myoglobin

318. Besides hemoglobin, there are other proteins that reversibly bind O_2. Regarding to them, which of the following assertions is true?

a. myoglobin acts as an O_2 storage in the muscle of mammals. As hemoglobin, it's formed by 4 subunits and the binding of O_2 is cooperative
b. eritrocruorins are giant proteins, with many heme groups, that transport O_2 in the blood of annelids
c. leghemoglobin is found in root nodules of legumes. It has a greater affinity for O_2 than hemoglobin, and allows a high concentration of O_2 within the nodule, thus allowing the plants to fix N_2
d. hemerythrin contains heme groups and Fe^{2+}, and transports O_2 in some marine invertebrates
e. hemocyanin transports O_2 in the blood of molluscs and arthropods. It uses prosthetic groups that bind Cu^+ and adopts an intense red colour when it is in contact with O_2

319. Hemoglobin...

a. is present in all vertebrates
b. is present in all vertebrates but in crocodile icefishes, that are some fishes which live in very cold waters
c. increases the level of O_2 in blood of mammals, approximately until the double concentration that it would be in pure water at the same temperature an pH
d. has not been detected until now in invertebrates
e. has not been detected until now in animals that breathe through gills

320. Which of the following assertions is FALSE?

a. Leghemoglobin has greater affinity for O_2 than hemoglobin.
b. The presence of free O_2 in the roots of legumes increases their ability to fix N_2.
c. Leghemoglobin avoids the inhibition of O_2 sensitive nitrogenase (the one that fixes atmosferic N_2).
d. Leghemoglobin has to achieve a given concentration of O_2 in the nodule, enough for the bacteria of the genus *Rhizobium* to breathe, but not excessive since nitrogenase must not be inhibited.
e. Leghemoglobin can transport O_2 or N_2.

321. Which of the following assertions is TRUE?

a. Each hemocyanin molecule binds two Cu^{2+} atoms, that are transformed into Cu^+ after binding O_2.
b. Hemocyanin, when bound to O_2, as many Cu^{2+} compounds in solution, adopts an intense red colour.
c. Hemocyanins, in hemolymph of molluscs and arthropods, are transported within cells, in the same way than hemoglobin is transported by the erythrocytes of mammals.
d. Cu^+/Cu^{2+} atoms are directly bound to hemocyanins by means of histidine residues. These lateral chains anchor methals, so they could bind O_2, in a similar function to that of heme groups in vertebrates.
e. Hemocyanins generally function in a monomeric form. Each monomer contains two cupper atoms.

322. In relation to myoglobin, which of the following assertions is FALSE?

a. Each molecule of myoglobin has a unique heme group covalently attached. It is essential for the binding of Fe^{2+} and O_2.
b. Is the protein responsible for the reddish colour of vertebrate musculature.
c. Its 3D structure was determined at the end of the decade of 1950 by John Kendrew.
d. Is mainly constituted by 8 hélices α-helices, each one bearing an heme group that can bind two Fe^{2+} atoms.
e. Raw meat is reddish since the most of the myoglobin has iron in its reduced form (Fe^{2+}). At high temperatures, meat adopts the brown colour typical of cooked meat, since iron atoms are mainly oxidized (Fe^{3+}).

323. The difference between heme A and B groups is...

a. A has an isopreneid added in the β position of one of the pyrrole rings
b. A has two carboxylic groups (-COOH) added in the β position of two apposite pyrrole rings
c. B has a larger molecular weight than A
d. A is more abundant, since it is present in hemoglobin
e. B has 5 pyrrole rings, thus its binding to Fe^{2+} is stronger

324. Which of the following assertions related to blood coagulation is FALSE?

a. Intrinsic pathway includes the activation of XII factor or Hageman's factor
b. The absence of VIII factor is the main reason for classic hemophilia
c. After a vessel injury, the release of tissular factor triggers the beginning of extrinsic pathway
d. X factor activation requires factors IX and VIII
e. Plasmin, derived from plasminogen proteolysis, strengthens adhesion between fibrin molecules forming the clot.

325. Which of the following assertions on heme groups is TRUE?

a. heme group A, besides hemoglobin, can be found in inflammation involved proteins such as COX-1 and COX-2
b. heme group A is found in membrane bound cytochromes
c. heme group A is the most abundant heme group in vertebrates
d. heme group B binds hemoglobin by non-covalent bonds mainly driven by 2 tyrosine residues
e. COX-1 and COX-2 proteins do not have heme groups

326. Identify the following molecules

a. A (heme A), B(heme B), C (heme C), D (porphyrin)
b. A (heme B), B(heme A), C (heme C), D (porphyrin)
c. A (heme A), B(heme B), C (porphyrin), D (heme C)
d. A (heme C), B(heme B), C (porphyrin), D (heme A)
e. A (heme A), B(heme C), C (porphyrin), D (heme B)

327. In the binding of O_2 to hemoglobin...

a. it's bound only a molecule of O_2 for each heme group, since the other locus of binding to Fe^{2+} is forming a H-bond with an histidine residue

b. it's bound a molecule of O_2 to each one of the two loci of coordination of Fe^{2+}, being it transformed to Fe^{3+}

c. other small molecules, as CO_2 (carbon dioxide), CO (carbon monoxide), or NO (nitric oxide), can also bind to Fe^{2+} with an affinity slightly lower than that of O_2

d. serine and threonine residues alternate to protect the second coordination site of Fe^{2+} against the binding of a second O_2

e. both distal histidine and bound O_2 access to the heme group from face of the porphyrine ring

328. Among the following molecules...

a. A is heme B, and B is heme O. Both groups associate to oxidase proteins

b. C is the heme O, present in bacteria, associated to oxidase proteins

c. B is heme C, present bc_1 complex, in the electronic transport chain

d. B is heme B, heme group is the most abundant, present in hemoglobin and also named protoporphyrin IX when it has not Fe^{2+} bound

e. D is heme C, also named protoheme IX

329. Blood rich in O_2 presents a hotter red colour than the blood poor in O_2, that is darker. This is because...

a. hemoglobin, when it has O_2 bound, is multimeric and has a hotter colour than when it has not O_2 bound, that is monomeric

b. the binding of O_2 to Fe^{2+} modifies the electronic properties of the porphyrine ring and this generates the change in colour

c. the binding of O_2 to the histidine in the active site of hemoglobin changes the electronic properties of this aromatic residue and a color change is caused

d. solution of Fe^{3+} have generally a hotter colour than solutions of Fe^{2+}. After the binding of O_2 to Fe^{2+}, iron is transformed to Fe^{3+} and a color change is caused

e. in the blood without O_2, hematocrit is higher, which indicates a higher amount of cells and an increase in the density of the fluid. Is for this reason that we see blood darker.

330. CO is toxic for aerobic organisms ...

a. since it oxidizes the OH groups of hemoglobin, avoiding this protein to fix O_2 properly

b. since it enters mitochondria, collecting the electrons of transport chain with lower efficiency than O_2

c. since it binds to heme group with higher affinity than O_2

d. since it prevents proximal histidine, in the active site of haemoglobin, from forming a H-bond with Fe^{2+}

e. since, as having a higher dipolar character, it is more soluble than O_2 in the blood, thus blocking the interchange of O_2 between air and blood at the level of pulmonary alveoli

331. CO...

a. has a lower affinity than O_2 for hemoglobin

b. has twice the affinity of O_2 for hemoglobin

c. has 2.500 times more affinity than O_2 for hemoglobin

d. has 25.000 times more affinity than O_2 for hemoglobin

e. has 250 times more affinity than O_2 for hemoglobin

332. Carboxyhemoglobin...

a. is an hemoglobin that presents heme group of type A, in which a pyrrole ring is substituted by an isopreneid chain
b. is a form of hemoglobin oxidized in the β carbons of the four pyrrole rings
c. is the form of hemoglobin reversibly bound to carbon monoxide
d. is hemoglobin when heme group is empty
e. is a type of hemoglobin in which proximal histidine has been substituted by aspartic acid or glutamic acid, being the carboxylic groups of these amino acids the ones that form H-bond with Fe^{2+}

333. Which of the following assertions is TRUE?

a. Carboxyhemoglobin blood levels, for a healthy person, are between 0.01 and 0.05% of total hemoglobin
b. Carboxyhemoglobin blood levels, for a healthy person, are around 0.1% of total hemoglobin. In smokers, these values usually triple, reaching the 3% in extreme cases.
c. Carboxyhemoglobin blood levels, for a healthy person, are around 1% of total hemoglobin. In smokers, these values are between 3 and 8%, reaching 30% in extreme cases.
d. For an average person (75 kg and 175 cm), to exceed a level of 5% of carboxyhemoglobin means enter in a coma.
e. Carboxyhemoglobin levels for a smoker are within the range of values for non-smoker people.

334. Fe^{2+} has an octahedric coordination ...

a. ...which means that it must have 6 ligands bound to it
b. ...which means that it must have 8 ligands bound to it
c. ...which means that it must have 10 ligands bound to it
d. ...which means that it must have 12 ligands bound to it
e. ...which means that it must have 20 ligands bound to it

335. The following table relates blood carboxyhemoglobin levels with the most usual symptoms. Indicate which of the columns does contain the right values (all them are values measured in non-smoker people, that do not suffer from any lung or heart disease, circumstances that would make the ranges to vary).

CARBOXYHEMOGLOBIN LEVELS (%of total hemoglobin)					SYMPTOMS
A	B	C	D	E	
0-0.1	0-10	0-5	0-0.1	0-0.1	Non detectable symptoms
0.1-10	10-20	5-15	0.1-2	0.1-2	Mild headache
10-20	20-50	15-30	2-10	2-20	Intense headache, sickness, giddiness, disorientation, visual disorders,...
>20	>50	>30	>10	>20	Coma
>30	>60	>40	>20	>30	Death

a. A
b. B
c. C
d. D
e. E

336. Which of the following assertions is FALSE?

a. If we are in a place with excess of CO in air, the more exercise we do, the higher the increase of carboxyhemoglobin concentration in blood
b. If we are in a place with excess of CO in air, the larger time we are exposed to this gas, the higher the increase of carboxyhemoglobin concentration in blood
c. If we are in a place with excess of CO in air, generally the increase of carboxyhemoglobin concentration in blood will not make us to show poisoning symptoms unless it exceeds 10%
d. Fetal hemoglobin fetal has a lower affinity for CO than adult hemoglobin, thus fetus are slightly more protected against CO poisoning
e. Normal levels of CO in the atmosphere are in the range from 0.05 to 4 ppm. In work areas where workers stay around 8 hours, a recommended standard is do not exceed 50 ppm

337. Which of the following assertions is FALSE?

a. CO, when binding an haemoglobin monomer, increases the affinity of the three other monomers for O_2
b. CO binds also other proteins different of hemoglobin
c. Binding of a CO molecule to an hemoglobin molecule complicates the transfer of O_2 from haemoglobin to tissues
d. If carboxyhemoglobin blood concentration is of 50%, the effects on O_2 distribution to tissues are equivalent to those found in an anemic person with haemoglobin levels reduced to half of its normal value
e. CO can be tightly bound to hemoglobin and haemoglobin can transport O_2 at the same time

338. P_{450} cytochromes share a common structural characteristic, which is it?

a. ...6 α-helices surround the heme group
b. ...the two positions of heme group not bound to porphyrin are occupied by aspartate residues, that leave this site in the presence of O_2 or carbon monoxide, to allow the coordination of these gases
c. ...one of the coordination positions of heme group constitutively binds an ionized cupper atom (Cu^{2+}), which generates that these proteins strongly absorb light at 450 nm
d. ...one of the six coordination positions of heme group is occupied by a thiolate ion of a cysteine
e. ...they present 4 hydroxyproline residues covalently attached to heme group

339. Which of the following assertions is FALSE?

a. The pressure of O_2 in lung air is higher than that found in tissues
b. The pressure of O_2 in lung air is in the range of 10-14 kPa
c. The pressure of O_2 in the tissues is in the range of 3-5 kPa
d. At high O_2 pressures (>12 kPa) the saturation level of hemoglobin by O_2 is similar for the following two cases. 1) an anemic person that has haemoglobin level reduced to the half of its normal value; 2) a person of the same dimensions with the level of carboxyhemoglobin in blood about 50%
e. At low O_2 pressures (<4 kPa) the saturation level of hemoglobin by O_2 is similar for the following two cases. 1) an anemic person that has haemoglobin level reduced to the half of its normal value; 2) a person of the same dimensions with the level of carboxyhemoglobin in blood about 50%

340. Fe²⁺ has an octahedric coordination. This means that the structure formd by Fe²⁺ and its ligands is represented by figure...

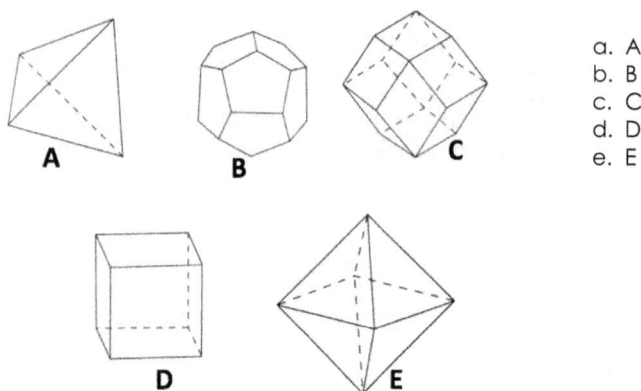

a. A
b. B
c. C
d. D
e. E

341. We name oximyoglobin...

a. ...to the myoglobin that has covalently bound an O_2 molecule
b. ...to the myoglobin that has bound an O_2 molecule in a non-covalent way
c. ...to the myoglobin that has covalently bound an O atom
d. ...to the myoglobin that has bound an O atom in a non-covalent way
e. ...to the myoglobin that has H-bond acceptor groups of distal histidine (-N-atoms) covalently binding an O_2 molecule

342. In myoglobin, proximal histidine, directly bound to Fe²⁺, is the residue number ...

a. 56
b. 61
c. 82
d. 93
e. 105

343. In oximyoglobin, distal histidine, directly bound to O_2, is the residue number...

a. 64
b. 74
c. 84
d. 94
e. 104

344. In myoglobin, proximal histidine, directly bound to Fe^{2+}, is in the helix ...

a. D
b. F
c. A
d. H
e. C

345. In oximyoglobin, distal histidine, directly bound to O_2, is in the helix...

a. E
b. H
c. I
d. C
e. A

346. In myoglobin, proximal histidine, directly bound to Fe^{2+}, is...

a. the residue 13 of helix F
b. the residue 8 of helix F
c. the residue 36 of helix F
d. the residue 44 of helix F
e. the residue 65 of helix F

347. In oximyoglobin, distal histidine, directly bound to O_2, is ...

a. the residue 12 of helix F
b. the residue 7 of helix F
c. the residue 35 of helix F
d. the residue 43 of helix F
e. the residue 64 of helix F

348. In oximyoglobin, O_2 molecule directly binds ...

    a. distal histidine (His 64) and proximal histidine (His 93)
    b. two pyrrole rings opposite to heme group
    c. Fe^{2+} atom and one of the N atoms of proximal histidine (His 93)
    d. Fe^{2+} atom anchored in the center of heme group and distal histidine (His 64)
    e. two pyrrole rings adjacent to heme group

349. In aqueous solution, the contact of Fe^{2+} with O_2 produces the oxidation of this metal to Fe^{3+}. The fact that Fe^{2+} is bound to heme group does not avoid this reaction. Why, in myoglobin, Fe^{2+}, O_2 and protein can remain together without the oxidation of Fe^{3+} being produced?

    a. since active site is a very hydrophobe environment
    b. since distal histidine oxidizes when O_2 binds
    c. since proximal histidine oxidizes when O_2 binds
    d. since heme group would reduce iron if it was oxidized to Fe^{3+}
    e. because Fe^{2+} participates of electron conjugated system of heme group, gaining electrons when they are needed, being very difficult its oxidation

350. If hemoglobin (or myoglobin) is stored in direct contact with air, iron is slowly oxidized forming metahemoglobin (o metamyoglobin). In these circumstances...

    a. O_2 binding site saturates by excees of O_2, and only competitive agonists with high affinity, like CO, can bind there
    b. the high partial pressure of O_2 (21% in atmospheric air) allows the formation of covalent bonds between O_2 and Fe^{2+}, that inactivate the binding site in a practically irreversible way
    c. the access of small molecules to O_2 binding site is complicated by a conformational change, and so hemoglobin gets inactivated
    d. the affinity of heme group for O_2 is reduced, heme pyrrole rings are protonated and the active site loses its ability to bind O_2
    e. O_2 binding site its inactivated and, in the place of this gas, a molecule of water is bound

351. Hemoglobin (or myoglobin)...

    a. allows the binding of O_2 and the oxidation of Fe^{2+}
    b. allows the binding of O_2 and the reduction of Fe^{2+}
    c. allows the binding of O_2, but not the oxidation of Fe^{2+}
    d. allows the O_2, while it's transported, to oxidize Fe^{2+} to Fe^{3+}, for this Fe^{3+} to be transferred to some specific cell types (i.e. glial cells)
    e. allows the binding of O_2, with the corresponding oxidation of heme group and its derivation towards the synthesis of bile salts

352. Which of the following structures does correspond to hemoglobin?

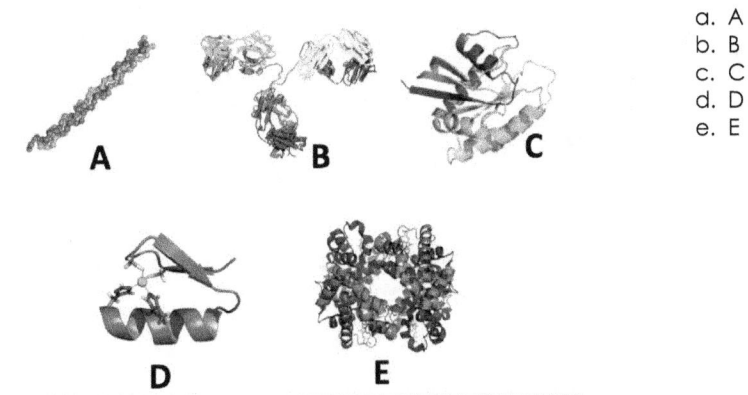

a. A
b. B
c. C
d. D
e. E

353. Which of the following assertions on O_2 and CO characteristics is FALSE?

a. molecular weight of CO is slightly lower
b. O_2 has a lower solubility in water than CO
c. O_2 is more abundant than CO in air
d. O_2 acts as a final electron acceptor in the aerobic metabolism
e. CO can cause poisoning by inhalation

354. Which of the following assertions is right?

a. human body produces CO, for instance in the reaction for degrading heme groups, thus a 1% of the binding sites of O_2 to hemoglobin are blocked in normal conditions
b. human body normally captures small amounts of CO by breathing. This, besides endogenous CO production, causes that a 10% of the binding sites of O_2 to hemoglobin are blocked in normal conditions
c. cells do not produce CO, it is a gas incorporated to cells from outside
d. in normal conditions, CO present in blood, regardless of its origin, binds to hemoglobin, saturating about a 10% of O_2 binding sites
e. in normal conditions, CO present in blood, regardless of its origin, binds to hemoglobin, triggering the separation of monomers and causing about a 10% of this protein to be useless for O_2 binding

355. Which of the following structures does correspond to myoglobin?

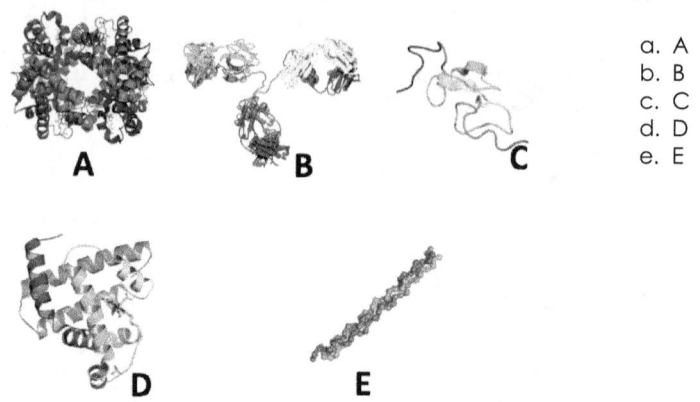

a. A
b. B
c. C
d. D
e. E

356. Which is the right assertion?

a. affinity of isolated ferroporphyrins (i.e. heme group not bound to hemoglobin) for the binding of CO is 25.000 times higher than for the binding of O_2
b. affinity of isolated ferroporphyrins (i.e. heme group not bound to hemoglobin) for the binding of CO is 10 times higher than for the binding of O_2
c. affinity of isolated ferroporphyrins (i.e. heme group not bound to hemoglobin) for the binding of CO is 200 times higher than for the binding of O_2
d. affinity of isolated ferroporphyrins (i.e. heme group not bound to hemoglobin) for the binding of CO is 200 times lower than for the binding of O_2
e. isolated ferroporphyrins do not bind O_2 nor CO

357. Indicate the true assertion...

a. affinity of hemoglobin to bind CO is 25.000 times higher than to bind O_2
b. affinity of hemoglobin to bind CO is 10 times higher than to bind O_2
c. affinity of hemoglobin to bind CO is 200 times higher than to bind O_2
d. affinity of hemoglobin to bind CO is 200 times lower than to bind O_2
e. affinity of hemoglobin to bind CO is 10 times lower than to bind O_2

358. CO...

a. is a poisonous gas since it desestabilizes the formation of hemoglobin tetramers and blocks breathing
b. is a poisonous gas since it occupies the binding sites of O_2 to hemoglobin thus blocking breathing
c. is a poisonous gas since it reduces pH within lung alveoli, complicating gas interchange and blocking breathing
d. is a poisonous gas since its solubility in the blood is much higher than that of O_2
e. is a poisonous gas since it causes the aggregation of haemoglobin tetramers, forming insoluble complexes and thus blocking breathing

359. One of the following proteins is the most abundant (measuring the abundance in mass %) in the tissues of the majority of vertebrates. Which is?

a. collagen
b. elastin
c. fibronectin
d. albumin
e. hemoglobin

360. Vitamin C...

a. is a cofactor of the enzyme that catalyzes proline hydroxylación in collagen fibers
b. is a cofactor of the enzyme that catalyzes the formation of desmosine in elastin fibers
c. is essential for the process of O_2 binding to the heme group of muscular myoglobin
d. is an energetic substrate of citrate synthase in osseous tissue
e. none of the previous assertions is right

361. In the tissues that need mechanical resistance or hardness, collagen is very abundant. On the other hand, the tissues that require to function to be elastic have an structural protein very characteristic named...

a. elicidin
b. elastin
c. hookein
d. fibronectin
e. dynein

362. GroEL and GroES proteins are...

a. transporters of cholesterol and other lipids
b. chaperones
c. HIV proteases
d. antibodies
e. pancreatic phosphatases

363. Actin can be in a polymerized form (actin F) or in a globular form (actin G). Actin G monomers, to polymerize, need...

a. ...the binding of a cofactor named riboflavin
b. ...ATP binding
c. ...the binding of myosin
d. ...the binding of a cofactor named vitamin D
e. ...the binding of vitamin C

364. In actin F filaments, actin G monomers are arranged...

a. forming a single chain helix very rigid
b. forming a single chain helix very flexible
c. forming a double chain helix
d. forming a triple chain helix
e. forming tetramers that are finally stacked as something like a 4-chain helix

365. Actin filaments have a – end and a + end. Which of the following assertions in relation to this property is TRUE?

a. Polymerization rate is higher in + end
b. Despolymerization rate is higher in + end
c. Polimerization rate is lower in + end
d. Polymerization rate is higher in - end
e. Despolymerization rate is lower in - end

366. A myosin monomer is formed by 6 polypeptidic chains. Of them...

a. 1 is a heavy chain and 5 are heavy
b. 2 are heavy chains and 4 are light
c. 3 are heavy chains and 3 are light
d. 4 are heavy chains and 2 are light
e. 5 are heavy chains and 1 is light

367. Myosin long chains...

a. are structured in several β-sheets, that adopt a supersecondary structure known as β-barrel
b. are structured as 2 α helices that form a double chain helix between them
c. are structured as 3 α helices, slightly more packed than the canonical form, that constitute a triple helix similar to collagen helix
d. are structured in form of 2 β-sheets, that adopt a T-shaped supersecondary structure, in which both sheets remain perpendicular
e. are structured in a disordered way or random coil structure

368. Which of the following assertions is FALSE?

a. Digestion of myosin by trypsin produces two fragments: light meromyosin (LMM) and heavy meromyosin (HMM)
b. Heavy meromyosin has the light chains of myosin and tha binding site of myosin and actin
c. Heavy meromyosin fragmentation by papain produces S1 fragments (that contain binding site to actin) and S2 fragment
d. The action of papain allows the separation of the two myosin head domains
e. Different myosin chains usually form aggregates thanks to the high affinity between the S1 fragments of the different myosins

369. In muscle contraction mechanism, sarcomere shortens because...

a. ...myosin molecules walk on myosin molecules
b. ...actin molecules shorten
c. ...actin molecules dissolve and transform from polymeric to globular form
d. ...myosin molecules bind to ATP and so reduce their length
e. ...actin molecules strongly bind to tropomyosin and retract towards Z discs

370. The following figure represents 3D structure of a myosin head (globular region, also called S1 fragment, where actin binding occurs). In it there are 3 regions indicated. A region where we find myosin light chains (CHAINS region), other where ATP is bound (ATP region) and other where actin binds (BIND region). Which of the following options, regarding the location of these zones, is TRUE?

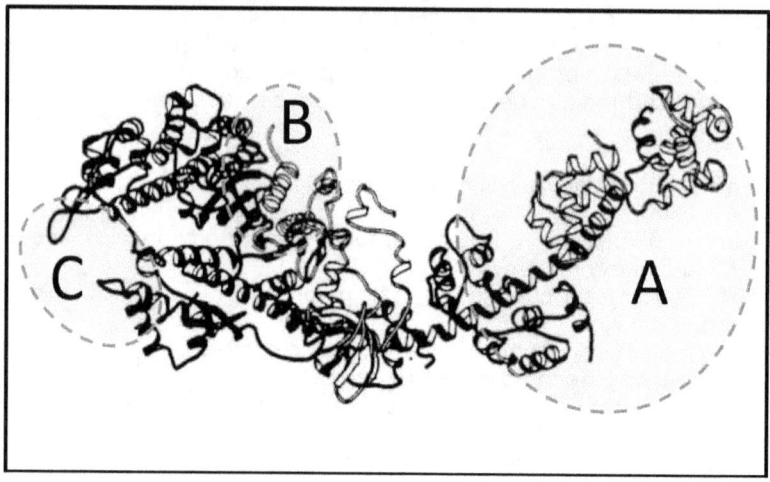

- a. A = BIND; B = ATP; C = CHAIN
- b. A = ATP; B = BIND; C = CHAIN
- c. A = CHAIN; B = BIND; C = ATP
- d. A = CHAIN; B = ATP; C = BIND
- e. A = ATP; B = CHAIN; C = BIND

371. Binding of ATP (and subsequent hydrolysis) to actin-myosin complexes within the sarcomere produces...

- a. a considerable reduction of pH
- b. a shortening of sarcomere
- c. the release of actin-myosin interaction
- d. actin polymerization
- e. the strengthening of actin-myosin interaction

372. Imagine the dynamics of contraction of a sarcomere. Each cycle initiates with myosin bound to actin. Subsequently, an ATP binds to myosin, and causes its separation from actin. A series of events happen later for the cycle to be closed:

A. Binding of Ca^{2+} to myosin
B. Binding of actin and myosin
C. ATP hydrolysis
D. Release of a group PO^{4-}

Order these events according to a chronological sequence

a. A → B → C → D
b. C → B → D → A
c. C → D → A → B
d. C → A → B → D
e. A → C → D → B

373. In the process of muscular contraction several proteins participate besides actin and myosin. One of them is a fibrous protein that arranges by forming extended dimers along the groove of actin F. It is...

a. Troponin I
b. Troponin C
c. Troponin T
d. Tropomyosin
e. Calcitonin

374. In the process of muscular contraction several proteins participate besides actin and myosin. One of them binds Ca^{2+} when its concentration rises, undergoes a conformational change and allows the formation of actin-myosin complexes. It is...

a. Troponin I
b. Troponin C
c. Troponin T
d. Tropomyosin
e. Calcitonin

375. In the process of muscular contraction several proteins participate besides actin and myosin. One of them binds to actin to maintain the complex actin-tropomyosin tightly bound, thus avoiding actin-myosin binding at low concentrations of Ca^{2+}. It does not bind Ca^{2+} when its concentration rises in the sarcomere, but it's sensitive to the conformational change generated when other protein binds Ca^{2+}. It is...

a. Troponin I
b. Troponin C
c. Troponin T
d. Tropomyosin
e. Calcitonin

376. In the process of muscular contraction several proteins participate besides actin and myosin. One of them is needed to maintain the complex actin-tropomyosin tightly bound, thus avoiding actin-myosin binding at low concentrations of Ca^{2+}. However, it does not directly bind actin. It does not bind Ca^{2+} when its concentration rises in the sarcomere, but it's sensitive to the conformational change generated when other protein binds Ca^{2+}. It is...

a. Troponin I
b. Troponin C
c. Troponin T
d. Tropomyosin
e. Calcitonin

377. In a generic microtubule of an eukaryotic cell, α and β isoforms of the protein tubulin combine approximately in a very characteristic proportion. Which is this proportion?

a. 10% of tubulin α and 90 % of tubulin β
b. 1/4 of tubulin α and 3/4 of tubulin β
c. the same amount of tubulin α and tubulin β
d. 3/4 of tubulin α and 1/4 of tubulin β
e. 90% of tubulin α and 10% of tubulin β

378. A microtubule has an external cylinder formed by a series of protofilaments, assembled in a parallel way. Each one is constituted by a series of alternated repeats of tubulin α and β. How many protofilaments do constitute the external cylinder of a microtubule?

  a. 12
  b. 13
  c. 14
  d. 15
  e. 16

379. A cilium has a basic cylindrical structure with ...

  a. 1 pair of central microtubules and 9 peripheral pairs
  b. 2 pairs of central microtubules and 12 peripheral pairs
  c. 1 pair of central microtubules and 15 peripheral pairs
  d. 1 pair of central microtubules and 12 peripheral pairs
  e. 2 pairs of central microtubules and 15 peripheral pairs

380. Which of the following lists does contain exclusively proteins that can be considered 'molecular motors' associated to microtubules?

  a. Keratin, lysonine, hemeritrine
  b. Myosin, lysine, estricmine
  c. Dynein, kinesin, nexin
  d. Dynamin, fibroin, collagen
  e. Sphingosine, cardiolipin, fibulin

Proteins: enzymology

381. A catalyst is a substance that...

a. ...easily dissolves in organic solvents, improving solvent fluidity, as occurs in engines that use unleaded petrol
b. ...accelerates the velocity of a chemical reaction
c. ...reduces the concentration of products in a chemical reaction
d. ...modifies thermodynamic equilibrium in a chemical reaction
e. ...reduces energy loss, specially when it comes to thermal energy, of a chemical reaction

382. An enzyme...

a. accelerates the velocity of a biochemical reaction because its active site is chemically complementary to reactives
b. accelerates the velocity of a biochemical reaction because its active site is chemically complementary to products
c. accelerates the velocity of a biochemical reaction because its active site is chemically complementary to the transition state of the chemical reaction
d. a, b and c are right
e. only a and b are right

383. The following graph is a Lineweaver-Burk representation for an enzymatic reaction. To which value does correspond the slope of the dashed line?

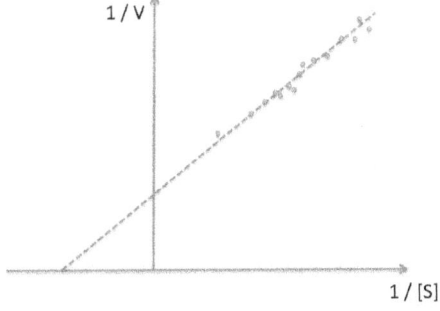

a. V_{max} / K_M
b. $1 / V_{max}$
c. K_M / V_{max}
d. $- V_{max} / K_M$
e. V_{max}

384. An enzyme that catalyzes the following chemical reaction, in which group (following the IUBMB enzyme commission rules) would be classified?

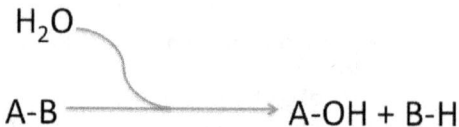

$$H_2O$$
$$A\text{-}B \longrightarrow A\text{-}OH + B\text{-}H$$

a. oxidoreductases
b. lyases
c. hydrolases
d. transferases
e. isomerases

385. Which of the following assertions is FALSE?

a. K_M measures the tendency of ES complex to dissociate
b. in a reaction following Michaelis-Menten kinetics, K_M is numerically equal to the concentration of substrate at which the velocity of reaction has reached half of its maximum value
c. if two enzymes have the same K_{cat}, the one that needs a lower concentration of substrate to reach $V_{max}/3$ is the one that has a lower K_M
d. K_{cat} is measured in moles/s
e. k_{cat} is the amount of substrate molecules that, when the enzyme functions at V_{max}, are converted into products in a second

386. The following graph is a Lineweaver-Burk representation for an enzymatic reaction. Which magnitudes are represented in X-Y axes?

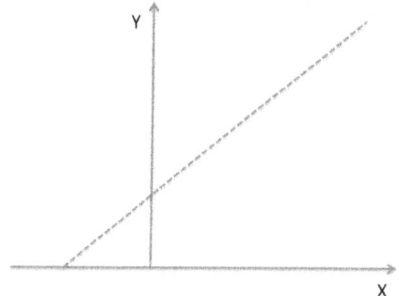

a. $X = [S] ; Y = V$
b. $X = 1/ [S] ; Y = 1 / V$
c. $X = 1 / V ; Y = 1 / [S]$
d. $X = V ; Y = [S]$
e. $X = 1 / V ; Y = [S]$

387. Trypsin...

a. ...catalyzes the binding of O_2 to transporting proteins (hemoglobin, leghemoglobin, hemocyanin,....)
b. ...catalyzes ATP hydrolysis actin-myosin junctions in muscle cells
c. ...catalyzes starch hydrolysis
d. ...catalyzes phosphorylation of some products of glycolysis (fructose-1,6bisP; glyceraldehyde-3-P;...)
e. ...catalyzes the breaking of peptide bond

388. What enzyme does catalyse the following reaction?

$$2 H_2O_2 \rightarrow 2 H_2O + O_2$$

a. Catalase
b. Oxygenase
c. Trypsin
d. Amylase
e. Myosin

389. Which of the following assertions is TRUE?

a. the relation K_{cat} / K_M is a measure of enzymatic efficiency
b. the product of V_{max} and [S] is a measure of enzymatic efficiency
c. the relation K_{cat} / [S] is a measure of enzymatic efficiency
d. the relation K_M / [S] is a measure of enzymatic efficiency
e. K_M is a measure of enzymatic efficiency

390. For any enzymatic reaction following Michaelis-Menten kinetics, K_M is numerically equal to...

a. ...the velocity at which the ES complex is dissociated
b. ...the velocity at which the ES complex is formed
c. ......the velocity at which the product of reaction is formed
d. ...the concentration of substrate at which the velocity of reaction has reached its maximum value
e. ...the concentration of substrate at which the velocity of reaction has reached half its maximum value

391. Which of the following assertions is FALSE?

a. A zymogen is a protein that is secreted in an inactive form, and needs to be proteolyzed to lead to the active enzyme.

b. Examples of zymogens are proelastase, trypsinogen, procarboxypeptidase and chymotrypsinogen.

c. Active trypsin catalyzes the formation of more active trypsin by proteolysis of trypsinogen.

d. Thrombin catalyzes the formation of fibrinogen clots by fibrin proteolysis.

e. Active trypsin generates elastase by proteolysis of proelastase.

392. The reaction...

$$2 H_2O_2 \rightarrow 2 H_2O + O_2$$

....is spontaneous but extremely slow in absence of a proper catalyst. In a tube of hydrogen peroxide we add a series of compounds. Which of them will accelerate the reaction in the most notable way?

a. Vertebrate's blood

b. A solution 0,1M of $FeCl_3$

c. A solution 0,1M of HCl

d. Cow's milk

e. An emulsion 0,1M of stearic acid in water

393. Catalase is an enzyme that catalyzes the following reaction:

a. Serine + ATP $\rightarrow$ Serine-P + ADP

b. $2 H_2O_2 \rightarrow 2 H_2O + O_2$

c. $CH_3COOH + O_2 \rightarrow 2 CO_2 + 2 H_2O$

d. 3 fatty acids + glycerol $\rightarrow$ triglyceride + H_2O

e. $C_6H_{12}O_6 + 6 O_2 \rightarrow 6 CO_2 + 6 H_2O$

394. Gluthatione peroxidase...

a. binds CO in erythrocytes at a rate that depends on gluthatione redox state

b. Oxidizes gluthatione, transforming it into three soluble amino acids, this reaction is generally coupled to the reduction of NAD^+ to NADH + H^+ although it can use NADPH

c. Oxidizes gluthatione. Normally it couples the reaction to the reduction of NAD^+ to NADH + H^+ although it can use NADPH

d. Catalyzes the oxidation of gluthatione coupled to the reduction of hydrogen peroxide to water

e. Catalyzes the reduction of gluthatione coupling it to hiperoxidation of alcohols, that in a high percentage gives rise to reactive oxygen species (ROS)

395. An enzyme that catalyzes the following chemical reaction, in which group (following the IUBMB enzyme commission rules) would be classified?

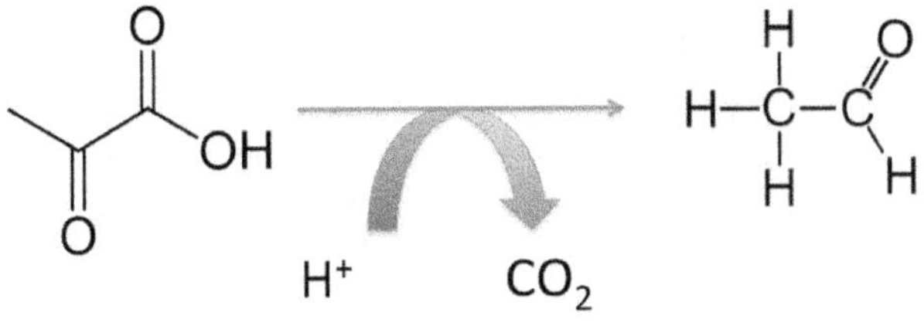

a. oxidoreductases
b. lyases
c. hydrolases
d. transferases
e. isomerases

396. An enzyme follows a Michaelis-Menten kinetics for the transformation of a given substrate S. Which of the following asserions is FALSE when it comes to the consequences of adding a competitive inhibitor to the process?

a. kinetics follow a Michaelis-Menten curve
b. velocity, for a given [S], is lower at velocities under V_{max}
c. V_{max} does not change
d. apparent K_M (K_M in presence of an inhibitor) is lower than K_M
e. velocity at which K_M is reached does not vary

397. The following graph is a Lineweaver-Burk representation for an enzymatic reaction. Which is the value of Y when the dashed line intersects with the Y-axis (the point indicated by the letter A)?

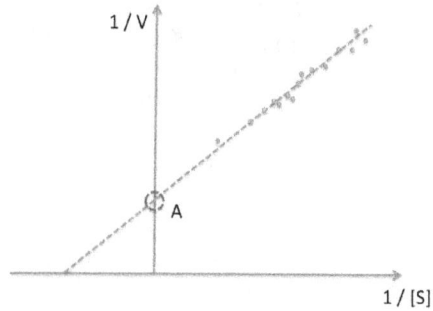

a. $1 / K_M$
b. $1 / V_{max}$
c. K_M
d. V_{max}
e. $-1 / K_M$

398. Diisopropylfluorophosphate (DFP) acts as an irreversible inhibitor of many proteins, such as acetylcholinesterase. Its mode of action is always the binding to an specific residue in the active site, always the same. Which is this residue?

a. serine
b. phenylalanine
c. histidine
d. lysine
e. aspartic acid

399. Chymotrypsin has a K_M of $1,5 \cdot 10^{-2}$ M and pepsin has a K_M of $3 \cdot 10^{-4}$ M. Which does need a higher concentration of substrate to reach an optimal catalysis velocity ($V_{max}/2$)?

a. chymotrypsin
b. pepsin
c. both need almost the same concentration of substrate
d. we can not determine it without knowing the K_{cat} of each enzyme
e. to reach $V_{max}/2$ substrate concentration would be the same, but to reach V_{max} pepsin will need a higher concentration

400. The following figure is an Eadie-Hofstee representation for an enzymatic reaction. Which magnitudes must be represented in the X-Y axes?

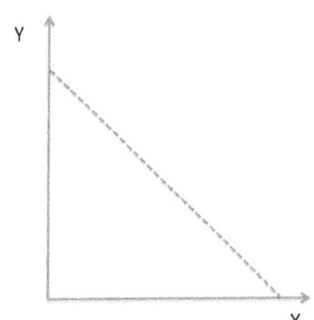

a. $X = [S]$; $Y = V$
b. $X = V$; $Y = V / [S]$
c. $X = V / [S]$; $Y = [S]$
d. $X = V$; $Y = [S]$
e. $X = V / [S]$; $Y = V$

401. The equation...

$$V = d[B]/dt$$

...expresses the velocity of a chemical reaction so simple as the irreversible conversion of A into B...

$$A \rightarrow B$$

...in terms of variation of product concentration in time. In which units is expressed the velocity (V) of this equation?

a. $mol \cdot s \cdot l^{-1}$
b. $mol \cdot s \cdot l^{-1}$
c. $mol \cdot s^{-1} \cdot l^{-1}$
d. $g \cdot s \cdot l^{-1}$
e. $g \cdot s \cdot l^{-1}$

402. We have an enzyme with a K_M of $2 \cdot 10^{-3}$ M for the substrate A. If $[A]_{initial}$ is of 10^{-5} M, and, after 1 minute of reaction, only a 2% of A has been transformed into product B. Which will be the [B] two minutes later?

a. $0,2 \cdot 10^{-5}$ M
b. $0,2 \cdot 10^{-6}$ M
c. $0,4 \cdot 10^{-6}$ M
d. $0,6 \cdot 10^{-6}$ M
e. $0,8 \cdot 10^{-6}$ M

403. An enzyme that catalyzes the following chemical reaction, in which group (following the IUBMB enzyme commission rules) would be classified?

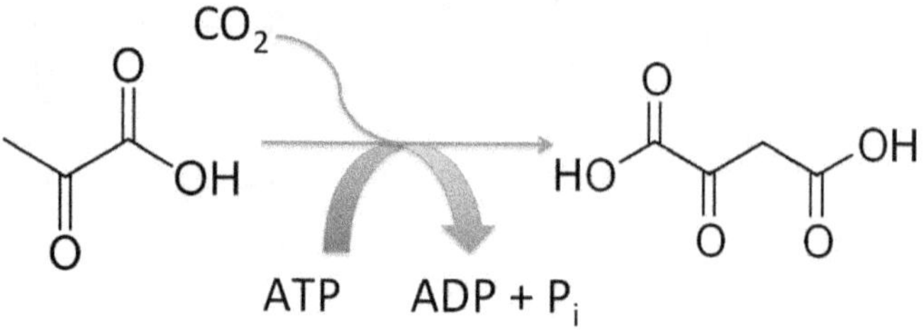

a. oxidoreductases
b. lyases
c. hydrolases
d. ligases
e. isomerases

404. We have an enzyme with a K_M of $2 \cdot 10^{-3}$ M for the substrate A. If $[A]_{initial}$ is of 10^{-5} M, and, after 1 minute of reaction only the 2% of A has been converted into the product B. Which is the V_{max} for this reaction at this enzyme concentration?

a. 10 μM/min
b. 40 μM/min
c. 70 μM/min
d. 100 μM/min
e. 130 μM/min

405. In the reaction...

A → B

...velocity of reaction is proportional to [A]. Proportionality constant is named k_1.

a. It is a first order reaction, when it comes to its kinetics
b. The higher the k_1, the higher the velocity of reaction
c. As [A] decreases, the velocity of the process is reduced
d. Velocity depends on the fisrt power of the concentration of the reactive, so it is a first order reaction
e. All the answers are right

406. Floretin hydrolase catalyzes the following hydrolysis reaction.

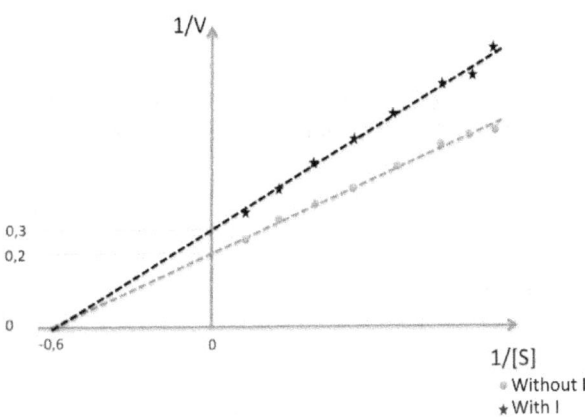

This enzymatic activity is assayed in presence of a non competitive inhibitor (I). The relation between the inverses of the velocity of reaction (V) and substrate concentration ([S]), is represented obtaining the following graph. Which is the V_{max}^{ap} for this enzyme in presence of the inhibitor?

a. -0.6
b. 0.2
c. 0.3
d. 3.33
e. 5

407. We want to calculate the inhibition constant (K_I) of a competitive inhibitor (I) of chymotrypsin. For this, enzymatic kinetics is evaluated at several concentrations of I. The following graph shows the relation between [I] and the different observed $K_M{}^{ap}$. Which is the value of K_M for chymotrypsin in absence of inhibitor?

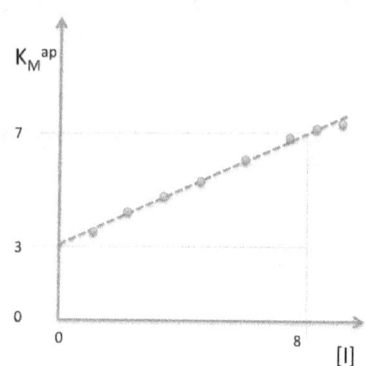

a. 0
b. 3
c. 4
d. 7
e. 8

408. Which of the following equations does correspond to the Michaelis-Menten equation? V_{max} = maximum velocity; K_M = Michaelis-Menten constant; V = reaction velocity; [S] = substrate concentration.

a. $V = (V_{max} \cdot [S]) / (K_M + [S])$
b. $V = (K_M + [S]) / (V_{max} \cdot [S])$
c. $V = (V_{max} + [S]) / (K_M \cdot [S])$
d. $V = (V_{max} + (1/[S])) / (K_M + [S])$
e. $V = [S] / (K_M + (V_{max} \cdot [S]))$

409. The following table shows the values of K_{cat} and K_M for the reaction of peptide bond breaking in a series of substrates catalysed by a synthetic protease. For which of the substrates is higher the specificity and efficiency of this enzyme?

Substrate	K_{cat}/K_M (M^{-1} s^{-1})
A	$6 \cdot 10^{-1}$
B	$1,2 \cdot 10^{-1}$
C	$1,6 \cdot 10^{2}$
D	$3,2 \cdot 10^{5}$

a. A
b. B
c. C
d. D
e. we can not know it with these data

146

410. The following figure is an Eadie-Hofstee representation for an enzymatic reaction. To which value does correspond the slope of the dashed line?

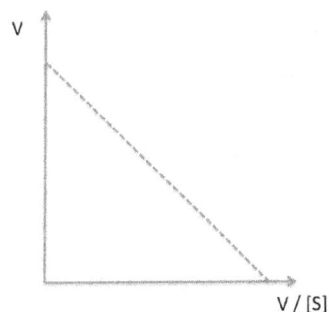

V / [S]

a. - K_M
b. K_M
c. V_{max}
d. $-V_{max}$
e. K_M/V_{max}

411. We have an enzyme with a K_M of $2 \cdot 10^{-3}$ M for the substrate A. If $[A]_{initial}$ is of 10^{-5} M, and, after 1 minute of reaction only the 2% of A has been converted into the product B. Which percentage of A would have reacted 3 after the beginning of the reaction?

a. 6 %
b. 10 %
c. 17 %
d. 23 %
e. more than 50 %

412. A commercial enzyme catalyzes the transformation of glucose-6-P into a fluorescent derivative. The K_M of this enzyme is $3 \cdot 10^{-4}$ M and V_{max} for this reaction is $1,5 \cdot 10^{-5}$ M. If we begin from a concentration of glucose-6-P of $9 \cdot 10^{-7}$ M, how long does it take for the 50% of glucose-6-P to react?

a. 3.2 min
b. 3.6 min
c. 6.8 min
d. 13.6 min
e. 22.2 min

413. The following figure is a **Lineweaver-Burk** representation for an enzymatic reaction. To which value does correspond the intersection of the dashed line with the X-axis, indicated with the letter A?

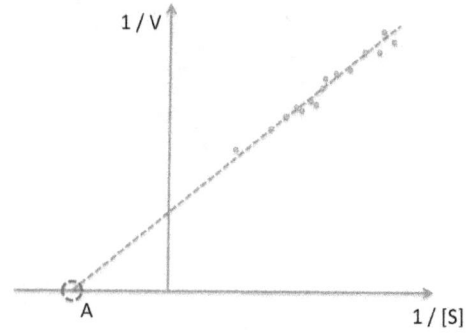

a. $1 / K_M$
b. $1 / V_{max}$
c. K_M
d. V_{max}
e. $-1 / K_M$

414. The following figure is an **Eadie-Hofstee** representation for an enzymatic reaction. To which value does correspond the intersection of Y-axis with the dashed line?

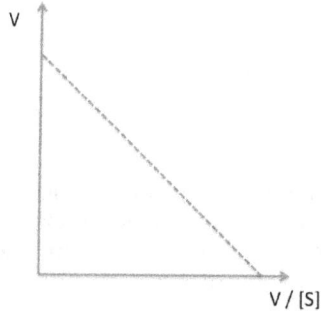

a. K_M
b. V_{max}/K_M
c. V_{max}
d. $-V_{max}$
e. K_M/V_{max}

415. A commercial enzyme catalyzes the transformation of glucose-6-P into a fluorescent derivative. The K_M of this enzyme is $3 \cdot 10^{-4}$ M and V_{max} for this reaction is $1.5 \cdot 10^{-5}$ M. If we begin from a concentration of glucose-6-P of 10^{-6} M, how long does it take for the 75% of glucose-6-P to react?

a. 0.2 min
b. 3.9 min
c. 10.4 min
d. 18.6 min
e. 27.2 min

416. We want to calculate the inhibition constant (K_i) of a competitive inhibitor (I) of chymotrypsin. For this, enzymatic kinetics is evaluated at several concentrations of I. The following graph shows the relation between [I] and the different observed K_M^{ap}. Which is the value of K_i?

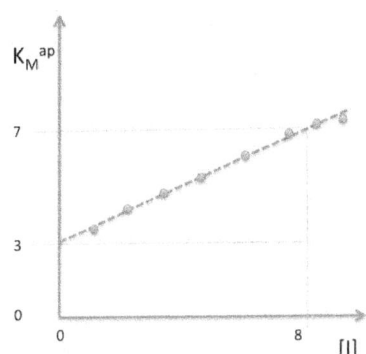

a. 0.5
b. 1.5
c. 2
d. 6
e. 8

417. We have an enzyme with a K_M of $2 \cdot 10^{-3}$ M for the substrate A. If $[A]_{initial}$ is of 10^{-5} M, and, after 1 minute of reaction only the 2% of A has been converted into product B. At which concentration of substrate will the V_{max} be reached?

a. 1 M
b. 0.6 M
c. 0.2 M
d. 0.9 M
e. 0.3 M

418. The enzyme β-diketone hydrolase participates in the reactions of alcoholic degradation of some fruits, catalysing the hydrolysis of 4,6-nonadione into pentan-2-one and butanoate. The K_M of this enzyme is of $1.2 \cdot 10^{-4}$ M. In only 30 s of reaction, a concentration of butanoate of 2.7 μM was obtained. Which will be the [butanoate] after 5.3 minutes from the beginning of the reaction?

a. $28.62 \cdot 10^{-6}$ M
b. $16.16 \cdot 10^{-6}$ M
c. $20.10 \cdot 10^{-5}$ M
d. $8.07 \cdot 10^{-6}$ M
e. $0.81 \cdot 10^{-4}$ M

419. The following figure is an **Eadie-Hofstee** representation for an enzymatic reaction. To which value does correspond the intersection of the dashed line with the X-axis?

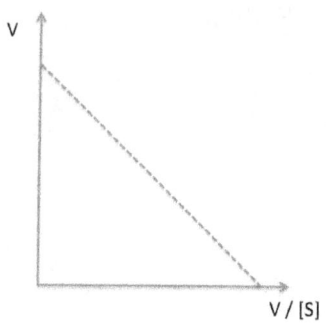

a. K_M
b. V_{max}/K_M
c. V_{max}
d. $-K_M$
e. K_M/V_{max}

420. The reaction catalysed by the enzyme cholesterol esterase follows, under normal conditions, a Michaelis-Menten kinetics. In the following experiment, the effect of crescent concentrations of two competitive inhibitors (I_a, I_b) in kinetic parameters was measured. The graph shows the relation between the concentration of each inhibitor and the K_M^{ap} of the reaction. Which is the value of K_M for cholesterol esterase without inhibitors?

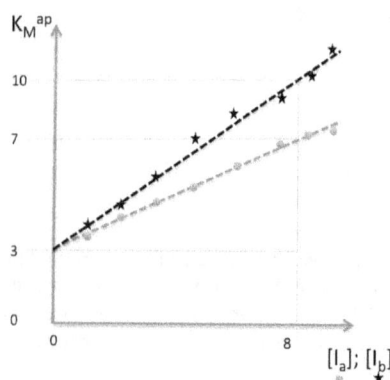

a. 0
b. 2
c. 3
d. 4
e. 8

421. The reaction catalysed by the enzyme cholesterol esterase follows, under normal conditions, a Michaelis-Menten kinetics. In the following experiment, the effect of crescent concentrations of two competitive inhibitors (I_a, I_b) in kinetic parameters was measured. The graph shows the relation between the concentration of each inhibitor and the $K_M{}^{ap}$ of the reaction. Which is the value of K_I for inhibitor a?

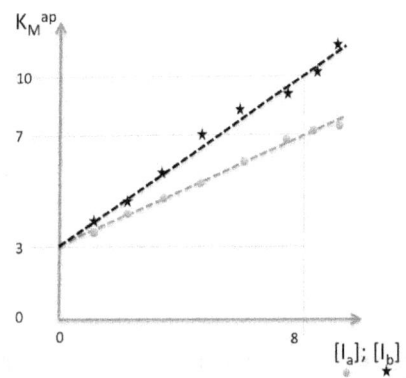

a. 0,5
b. 1,5
c. 2
d. 6
e. 8

422. An enzyme that catalyzes the following chemical reaction, in which group (following the IUBMB enzyme commission rules) would be classified?

a. oxidoreductases
b. lyases
c. hydrolases
d. ligases
e. isomerases

423. The reaction catalysed by the enzyme cholesterol esterase follows, under normal conditions, a Michaelis-Menten kinetics. In the following experiment, the effect of crescent concentrations of two competitive inhibitors (I_a, I_b) in kinetic parameters was measured. The graph shows the relation between the concentration of each inhibitor and the $K_M{}^{ap}$ of the reaction. Which is the value of K_i for inhibitor b?

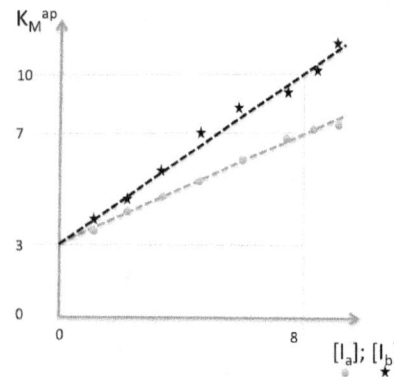

a. 0,38
b. 0,88
c. 2,63
d. 3,43
e. 7,00

424. Enzyme Comission (EC) of the International Union of Biochemistry and Molecular Biology (IUBMB) has proposed a naming system for classifying enzymes in 6 big groups. Which are these groups?

a. oxidoreductases, transferases, hydrolases, lyases, isomerases, ligases
b. oxidoreductases, polimerases, hydratases, lyases, isomerases, peptidases
c. oxidoreductases, transferases, hydrolases, lyases, isomerases, peptidases
d. oxidoreductases, transferases, hydrolases, maltases, isomerases, ligases
e. oxidoreductases, epimerases, hydrolases, lyases, polimerases, isomerases

425. Enzyme Comission (EC) of the International Union of Biochemistry and Molecular Biology (IUBMB) has proposed a naming system for classifying enzymes in 6 big groups. One of them is formed by oxidoreductases. Which type of reactions do they catalyse?

a. reactions in which two molecules are bound
b. intramolecular rearrangements
c. oxidation-reduction reactions
d. additions of a chemical group to a double bond
e. hydrolytic breakings

426. The activity of Isothiocyanate isomerase is assayed in presence of an inhibitor (I). We represent the relation between the inverses of the velocity of reaction (V) and of substrate concentration ([S]), obtaining the following graph. What is the value of the point indicated by the letter A?

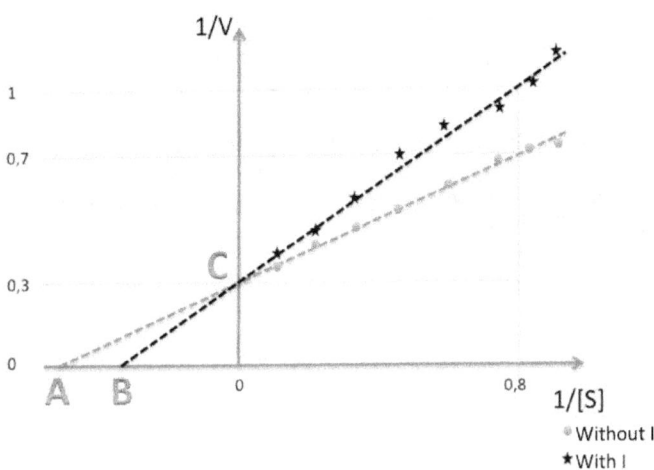

a. $1 / K_M$
b. $-1 / K_M$
c. $1 / V_{max}$
d. $1 / K_M{}^{ap}$
e. $-1 / K_M{}^{ap}$

427. An enzyme that catalyzes the following chemical reaction, in which group (following the IUBMB enzyme commission rules) would be classified?

a. oxidoreductases
b. lyases
c. hydrolases
d. ligases
e. isomerases

428. Floretin hydrolase catalyzes the following hydrolysis reaction.

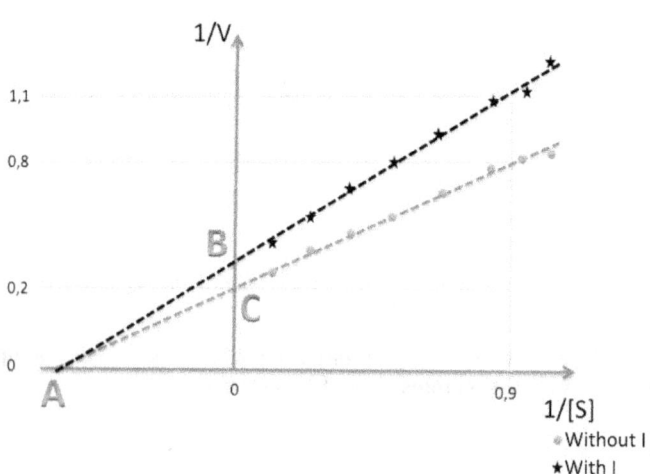

Floretin
hydrolase

This enzymatic activity is assayed in presence of a non-competitive inhibitor (I). The relation between the inverses of the velocity of reaction (V) and the concentration of substrate ([S]) is represented in the following graph. To which value does correspond the intersection indicated with the letter A?

a. $1 / K_M$
b. $-1 / K_M$
c. $1 / V_{max}$
d. $1 / K_M^{ap}$
e. $-1 / K_M^{ap}$

429. To calculate the inhibition constant (K_i) of a non-competitive inhibitor (I) of fumarase, we evaluate enzymatic kinetics at different concentrations of I. Relation between [I] and the different observed V_{max}^{ap} is represented in the following graph. Which is the value of K_i?

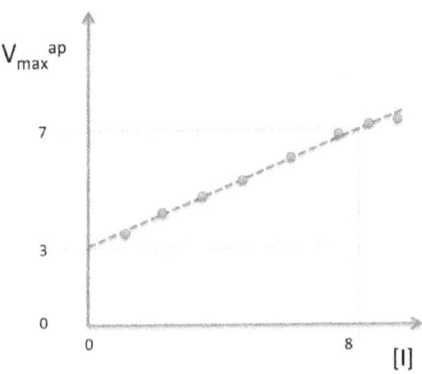

a. 0.17
b. 0.33
c. 0.67
d. 1.50
e. 6.00

430. Enzyme Comission (EC) of the International Union of Biochemistry and Molecular Biology (IUBMB) has proposed a naming system for classifying enzymes in 6 big groups. One of them is formed by ligases. Which type of reactions do they catalyse?

a. reactions in which two molecules are bound
b. intramolecular rearrangements
c. oxidation-reduction reactions
d. additions of a chemical group to a double bond
e. hydrolytic breakings

431. Enzyme Comission (EC) of the International Union of Biochemistry and Molecular Biology (IUBMB) has proposed a naming system for classifying enzymes in 6 big groups. One of them is formed by lyases. Which type of reactions do they catalyse?

a. reactions in which two molecules are bound
b. intramolecular rearrangements
c. oxidation-reduction reactions
d. additions of a chemical group to a double bond
e. hydrolytic breakings

432. The activity of Isothiocyanate isomerase is assayed in presence of an inhibitor (I). We represent the relation between the inverses of the velocity of reaction (V) and of substrate concentration ([S]), obtaining the following graph. What is the value of the point indicated by the letter B?

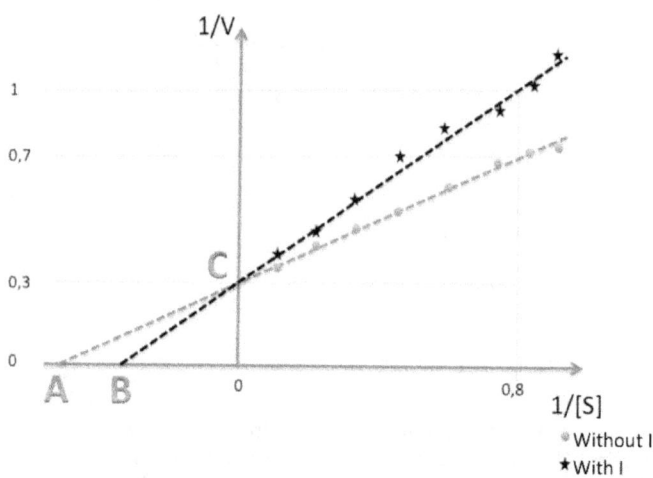

a. $1 / K_M$
b. $-1 / K_M$
c. $1 / V_{max}$
d. $1 / K_M{}^{ap}$
e. $-1 / K_M{}^{ap}$

433. Enzyme Comission (EC) of the International Union of Biochemistry and Molecular Biology (IUBMB) has proposed a naming system for classifying enzymes in 6 big groups. One of them is formed by hydrolases. Which type of reactions do they catalyse?

a. reactions in which two molecules are bound
b. intramolecular rearrangements
c. oxidation-reduction reactions
d. additions of a chemical group to a double bond
e. hydrolytic breakings

434. Floretin hydrolase catalyzes the following hydrolysis reaction.

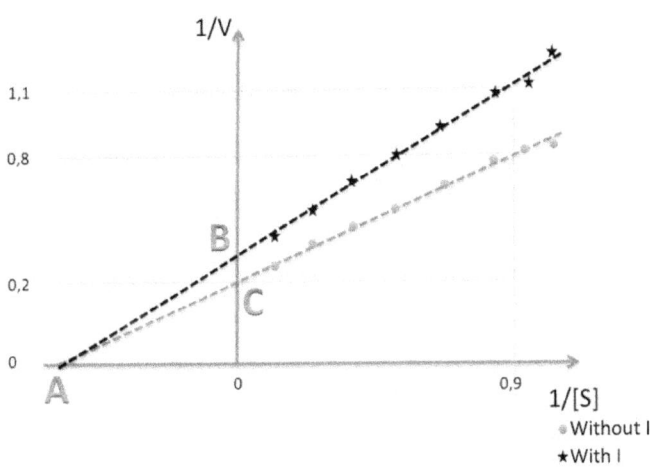

Floretin
hydrolase

This enzymatic activity is assayed in presence of a non-competitive inhibitor (I). The relation between the inverses of the velocity of reaction (V) and the concentration of substrate ([S]) is represented in the following graph. To which value does correspond the intersection indicated with the letter B?

a. $1 / V_{max}{}^{ap}$
b. $-1 / K_M$
c. $1 / V_{max}$
d. $1 / K_M{}^{ap}$
e. $-1 / K_M{}^{ap}$

435. Enzyme Comission (EC) of the International Union of Biochemistry and Molecular Biology (IUBMB) has proposed a naming system for classifying enzymes in 6 big groups. One of them is formed by isomerases. Which type of reactions do they catalyse?

a. reactions in which two molecules are bound
b. intramolecular rearrangements
c. oxidation-reduction reactions
d. additions of a chemical group to a double bond
e. hydrolytic breakings

436. The activity of Isothiocyanate isomerase is assayed in presence of an inhibitor (I). We represent the relation between the inverses of the velocity of reaction (V) and of substrate concentration ([S]), obtaining the following graph. What is the value of the point indicated by the letter C?

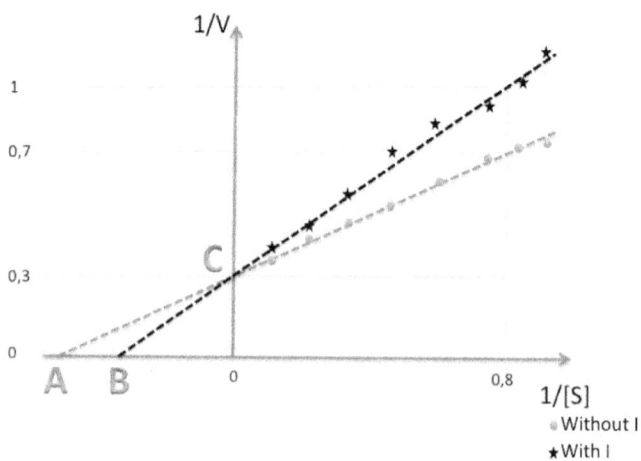

a. $1 / K_M$
b. $-1 / K_M$
c. $1 / V_{max}$
d. $1 / K_M^{ap}$
e. $-1 / K_M^{ap}$

437. A commercial enzyme catalyzes the transformation of glucose-6-P into a fluorescent derivative. A 10^{-6}M concentration of glucose reacts in presence of the enzyme and it's observed that 5% of the substrate reacts in 1 minute. If K_M of this enzyme is $3 \cdot 10^{-4}$ M, which is the value of V_{max}?

    a. 10^{-3} M·min^{-1}
    b. $0,5 \cdot 10^{-4}$ M·min^{-1}
    c. $1,5 \cdot 10^{-5}$ M·min^{-1}
    d. $3 \cdot 10^{-6}$ M·min^{-1}
    e. 10^{-4} M·min^{-1}

438. To calculate the inhibition constant (K_I) of a non-competitive inhibitor (I) of fumarase, we evaluate enzymatic kinetics at different concentrations of I. Relation between [I] and the different observed $V_{max}{}^{ap}$ is represented in the following graph. Which is the value of V_{max} for this enzyme in absence of the inhibitor?

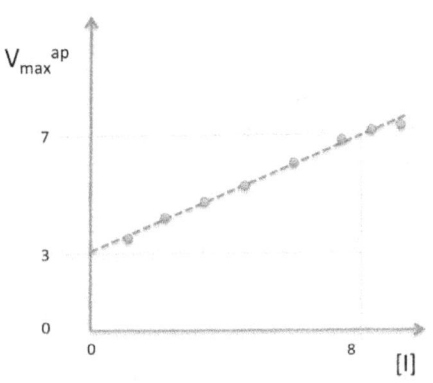

    a. 0,5
    b. 2
    c. 3
    d. 7
    e. 8

439. Michaelis-Menten constant (K_M) equals...

    a. ...the inverse of the concentration of substrate at the point where the velocity of reaction equals V_{max}
    b. ... the concentration of substrate at the point where the velocity of reaction equals V_{max}
    c. ... the inverse of the concentration of substrate at the point where the velocity of reaction equals (V_{max} / 2)
    d. ... the concentration of substrate at the point where the velocity of reaction equals (V_{max} / 2)
    e. ...none of the previous answers

440. We have an enzyme with a K_M of $2 \cdot 10^{-3}$ M for the substrate A. If $[A]_{initial}$ is 10^{-5} M, and after 1 minute of reaction only the 2% of A has been converted into the product B. Which would be the [A] 120 seconds later?

a. $8.2 \cdot 10^{-5}$ M
b. $9.4 \cdot 10^{-6}$ M
c. $0.1 \cdot 10^{-6}$ M
d. $4.5 \cdot 10^{-6}$ M
e. $11.8 \cdot 10^{-6}$ M

441. Floretin hydrolase catalyzes the following hydrolysis reaction.

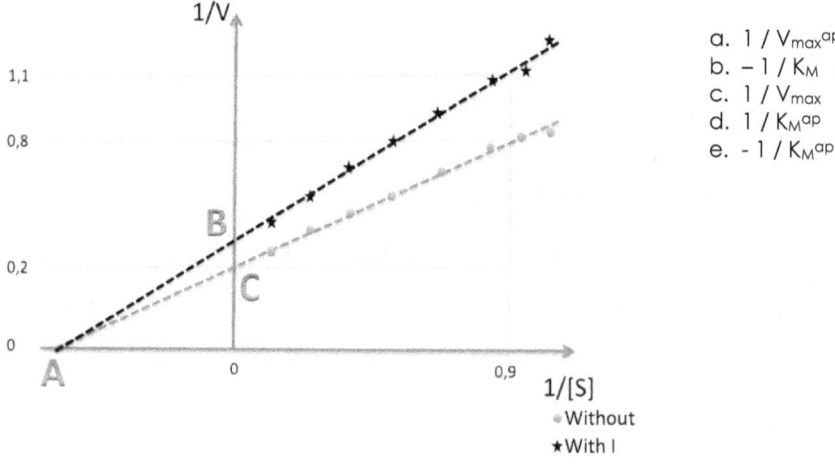

Floretin hydrolase

This enzymatic activity is assayed in presence of a non-competitive inhibitor (I). The relation between the inverses of the velocity of reaction (V) and the concentration of substrate ([S]) is represented in the following graph. To which value does correspond the intersection indicated with the letter C?

a. $1 / V_{max}{}^{ap}$
b. $-1 / K_M$
c. $1 / V_{max}$
d. $1 / K_M{}^{ap}$
e. $-1 / K_M{}^{ap}$

1/V

1,1

0,8

B

0,2

C

0

A

0

0,9

1/[S]

Without
With I

442. Floretin hydrolase catalyzes the following hydrolysis reaction.

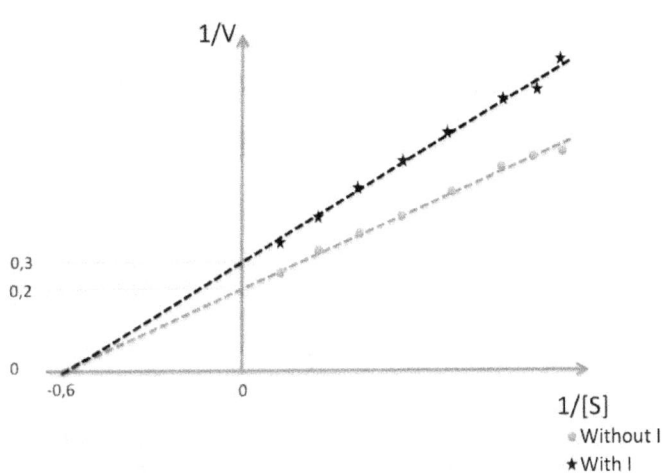

This enzymatic activity is assayed in presence of a non-competitive inhibitor (I). The relation between the inverses of the velocity of reaction (V) and the concentration of substrate ([S]) is represented in the following graph. Which is the V_{max} of this enzyme in the absence of inhibitor?

a. -0.6
b. 0.2
c. 0.3
d. 3.33
e. 5

443. Floretin hydrolase catalyzes the following hydrolysis reaction.

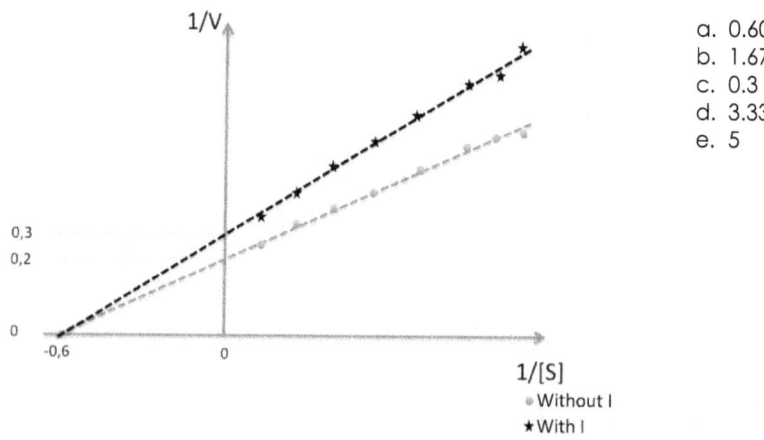

This enzymatic activity is assayed in presence of a non-competitive inhibitor (I). The relation between the inverses of the velocity of reaction (V) and the concentration of substrate ([S]) is represented in the following graph. Which is the K_M of this enzyme?

a. 0.60
b. 1.67
c. 0.3
d. 3.33
e. 5

444. A commercial enzyme catalyzes the transformation of glucose-6-P into a fluorescent derivative. A $10^{-6}M$ concentration of glucose reacts in presence of the enzyme and it's observed that 5% of the substrate reacts in 1 minute. Which percentage of substrate will react in 5 minutes. NOTE: the K_M of this enzyme is $3 \cdot 10^{-4}$ M

a. 23 %
b. 29 %
c. 35 %
d. 41 %
e. 48 %

Nucleotides and nucleic acids

445. The most frequent sugars in the nucleotides of living beings are...

a. β-D-xylulose and β-D-glucose
b. β-L-glucose and β-L-erythrose
c. β-D-ribose and β-D-deoxyribose
d. β-D-fructose and β-L-allose
e. β-D-trehalose and β-D-ribose

446. Identify the following structures corresponding to nitrogenous bases

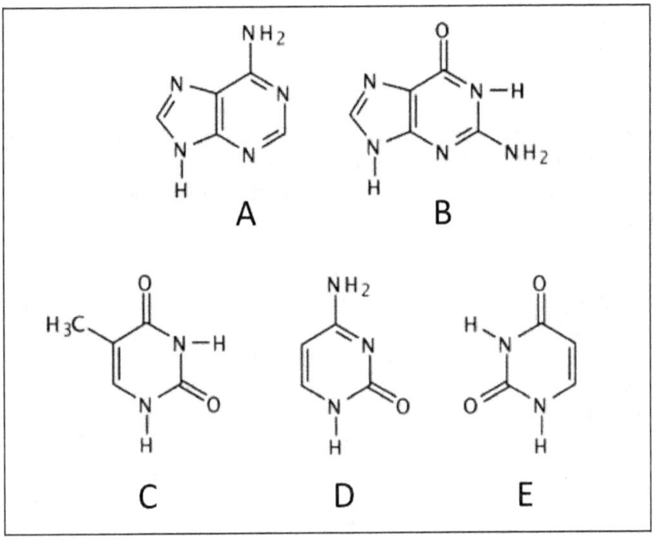

a. A=adenine; B=thymine; C=guanine; D=cytosine; E=uracil
b. A=adenine; B=guanine; C=thymine; D=cytosine; E=uracil
c. A=guanine; B=adenine; C=cytosine; D=uracil; E=thymine
d. A=guanine; B=adenine; C=uracil; D=cytosine; E=thymine
e. A=adenine; B=guanine; C=uracil; D=cytosine; E=thymine

447. In a codifying nucleotide, nitrogenous base binds to the sugar by...

a. ...a β-glycosidic bond
b. ...an α-glycosidic bond
c. ...an O-glycosidic bond of type β
d. ...an O-glycosidic bond of type α
e. ...a covalent carbon-carbon bond

448. In a nucleotide within DNA, thymine binds to carbon 1 β-D-deoxyribose by...

a. ...its carbon 6
b. ...its carbon 5
c. ...its nitrogen 3
d. ...its carbon 2
e. ...its nitrogen 1

449. One of the ways by which hydroxyl radicals are pathological is the generation of modified nucleobases, like 8-oxoguanine, isoguanine,... Why these modifications, that change chemical groups that do not participate directly in Watson Crick unions, are mutagenic?

a. Because they weaken sugar phosphate backbone and it breaks
b. Because these chemical modifications change the tautomeric preferences and the fidelity of nucleobases to the amino-oxo tautomers, allowing non-Watson Crick pairings that can originate transversions or transitions
c. Since dipoles of nucleobases are altered and the stacking interactions, which drive the selective preferences in Watson Crick pairings, are modified
d. Because the flexibility of sugar-base bond is strongly modified, allowing some conformations to prevail and form alternative pairings
e. Since the bases become much more soluble and DNA despolimerization is more favourable from a thermodynamic point of view

450. In a nucleotide within DNA, cytosine binds to carbon 1 of β-D-deoxyribose by...
a. ...its carbon 6
b. ... its carbon 5
c. ...its nitrogen 3
d. ... its carbon 2
e. ... its nitrogen 1

451. In nucleotides within DNA, phosphate group binds through esterification to two carbons, each one belonging to a different nucleotide in a pair of contiguous nucleotides. Which are these carbons?

   a. 4' and 3'
   b. 5' and 3'
   c. 1' and 2'
   d. 1' and 3'
   e. 1' and 4'

452. The most common H-bond donor groups in nucleobases are...

   a. N atoms within heterocyclic ring and O atoms of carbonile groups
   b. amine (-NH₂) and hydroxyl (-OH) groups hanging from heterocyclic ring
   c. hydroxyl (-OH) groups hanging from heterocyclic ring
   d. sp2 carbon atoms within heterocyclic rings
   e. amine groups (-NH₂)

453. In a nucleotide within RNA, thymine binds to carbon 1 of β-D-ribose by...

   a. ...its carbon 6
   b. ... its carbon 5
   c. ...its nitrogen 3
   d. ... its carbon 2
   e. ... its nitrogen 1

454. Canonical unions (Watson-Crick type) between adenine and thymine...

   a. involve a H-bond donor group of thymine and other donor group of adenine
   b. involve a a nitrogen atom as H-bond acceptor group in adenine, and an oxygen atom as acceptor group at thymine
   c. involve an oxygen atom as H-bond acceptor group in adenine, and a nitrogen atom as acceptor group at thymine
   d. a and b are right
   e. a and c are right

455. In a nucleotide within DNA, adenine binds to carbon 1 of β-D-deoxyribose by...

   a. ...its nitrogen 9
   b. ... its nitrogen 1
   c. ...its carbon 8
   d. ...its carbon 2
   e. ... its nitrogen 3

456. The most characteristic H-bond acceptor groups in nucleobases are...

a. the N atoms of heterocyclic ring and the O atoms of carbonyle groups
b. amine groups (-NH₂) and the hydroxyle groups (-OH) that hang from heterocyclic ring
c. the hydroxyle groups (-OH) that hang from the heterocyclic ring
d. the sp2 carbon atoms of heterocyclic rings
e. the amine groups (-NH₂)

457. The most frequent tautomeric forms of nucleobases within the DNA at pH=7 in aqueous solution are...

a. the forms keto-amino
b. the forms keto-imino
c. the forms enol-amino
d. the forms enol-imino
e. the forms enol-enamine

458. Stacking interactions between nucleobases...

a. are the ones established between the aromatic systems of two stacked nucleobases
b. are the ones established between the aromatic systems of any nucleobase and a cation
c. are the ones established between the aromatic systems of any nucleobase and an anion
d. are the ones established between the aromatic systems of any nucleobase and any charged particle
e. are the ones established between the aromatic systems of any nucleobase and a polar molecule (H₂O, NH₃,....)

459. The following picture represents the interaction between guanine and cytosine. Indicate what would be a Hoogsteen-type interaction for this system.

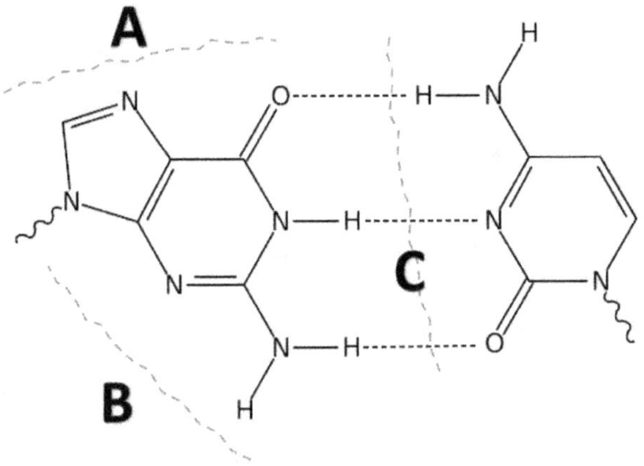

a. It's the interaction between any of the two bases and any aromatic heterocycle disposed in a paralle way in relation to the plane formed by both bases. They're also named 'stacking interactions'.
b. It's the interaction of any aromatic heterocycle with the bulkiest base (guanine in this case) being placed in a parallel way to the planed formed by this base. They're also named 'stacking interactions'.
c. It's the interaction of a third nucleobase through the face indicated with letter A, forming a coplanar triad.
d. It's the interaction of a third nucleobase through the face indicated with letter B, forming a coplanar triad.
e. It's the interaction of a third nucleobase through the face indicated with letter C, thus displacing the smallest nucleobase (cytosine in this case)

460. In a nucleotide within DNA, guanine binds to 1 of β-D-deoxyribose by...

a. ...its nitrogen 9
b. ...its nitrogen 1
c. ...its carbon 8
d. ...its carbon 2
e. ...its nitrogen 3

461. The most frequent DNA secondary structure is ...

    a. A-DNA
    b. B-DNA
    c. H-DNA
    d. T-DNA
    e. Z-DNA

462. Chargaff's rule establishes that...

    a. in a DNA fiber, the number of purine nitrogen bases is equal to the number of pyrimidine nitrogen bases
    b. the number of pyrimidine nitrogen bases in any nucleic acid (DNA, RNA,....) is directly proportional to the solubility of the fiber
    c. the number of purine nitrogen bases in a DNA fiber is directly proportional to the solubility of the fiber
    d. every pyrimidine nitrogen base is accompanied by a Na^+ cation in DNA, being also possible to find other cations (K^+, Mg^{2+},....) in other nucleic acid types
    e. every crystallized substance of which diffraction pattern shows a regular figure, has an helicoidal structure

463. In a B-type DNA double helix, the linear distance between a base-pair bound by H-bonds and the contiguous base-pair is about...

    a. 0.34 Å
    b. 0.34 mm
    c. 0.34 μm
    d. 0.34 nm
    e. 3.4 μm

464. The scientist _____ was the first to isolate DNA from _____.

    a. Erwin Chargaff / onion cells
    b. Matthew Messelson / mouse liver
    c. James Watson / porcupine quills
    d. Oswald Avery / *Drosophila* salivary glands
    e. Friedrich Miescher / salmon sperm

465. Between 1944 and 1952 the experiments of Avery, McLeod and McCarthy were developed. They quite clearly established that DNA was the material responsible for genetic information. In these experiments...

a. DNA of pathogenic lineages of *Pneumococcus* bacteria was transferred to non-pathogenic lineages, turning them into pathogenic

b. DNA was broken into its constituent monomers, concluding that it was formed by only four distinct monomers

c. DNA of pathogenic bacteria was labelled with ^{35}P, and by using optical microscopy it was observed how this DNA was transferred to non-pathogenic lineages, turning them into pathogenic

d. it was observed that, among the cells present in mouse blood cell cultures, only those with DNA in the nucleus (leukocytes) were able to divide, while erythrocytes or platelets did not divide

e. the concentration of DNA in bacterial cultures was measured (by spectrophotometry at a wavelength of 260 nm) and it was observed that such concentration increased proportionally with the number of cells present in the culture

466. The final proof that DNA was the genetic material was provided by Hershey and Chase experiment. They studied the infection of *Escherichia coli* bacteria by the T2 bacteriophage virus, by using radioactive labelling for the proteins (^{35}S) and the DNA (^{32}P) of the virus. In this experiment ...

a. ...infected bacteria produced T2 bacteriophage viruses, many of them with labelled DNA (^{32}P)

b. ...the proteins labelled by ^{35}S are also present in many of the bacteriophages produced by *Escherichia coli*

c. ...none of the bacteriophages produced by *Escherichia coli* contained ^{32}P

d. b and c are right

e. a and b are right

467. Watson and Crick model for DNA was a _____ helix, _____, with _____ base-pairs per turn.

a. triple / parallel / 7.5

b. double / antiparallel / 13

c. triple / antiparallel / 3.4

d. double / antiparallel / 10

e. double / antiparallel / 3.4

468. Watson and Crick, that were working at _____ University, had access to the fiber diffraction patterns obtained from concentrated DNA solutions photographed by _____, that was working in the laboratory of _____ at the _____ of London.

    a. Oxford / Irina Sarapova / Max Perutz / Max Planck Institute
    b. Bristol / Helena Ehrlich / Martha Chase / University College
    c. Leeds / Martha Chase / Alfred Hershey / Queen's College
    d. Londres / Marie Curie / Edward Jenner / Weizmann's Institute
    e. Cambridge / Rosalind Franklin / Maurice Wilkins / King's College

469. When comparing the chemical structure of an A-T pair (Watson-Crick type, that is, with both bases in the same plane and bound by H-bonds) with that of a G-C pair (also Watson-Crick type), the distance between C1' carbons of deoxyriboses...

    a. is higher for A-T pair (~1.5 nm) than for G-C pair (~0.7 nm)
    b. is higher for G-C pair (~1.5 nm) than for A-T pair (~0.7 nm)
    c. is approximately equal in both cases, being its value about ~1.1 nm
    d. is approximately equal in both cases, being its value about ~1.5 nm
    e. is approximately equal in both cases, being its value about ~0.7 nm

470. If we advance in 5'→3' direction in a DNA double helix...

    a. each base pair presents a rotation of ~3° in relation to the following pair
    b. each base pair presents a rotation of ~10° in relation to the following pair
    c. each base pair presents a rotation of ~15° in relation to the following pair
    d. each base pair presents a rotation of ~25° in relation to the following pair
    e. each base pair presents a rotation of ~36° in relation to the following pair

471. A-form of DNA is the most abundant...

    a. ...in the cell cytoplasm
    b. ...in the cell nucleus
    c. ...in low-salinity conditions
    d. ...in low-humidity conditions
    e. ...in the genome zones that are transcriptionally active

472. Some cell cultures grow in presence of several isotopes of nitrogen (^{15}N or ^{14}N). Next we measure the relative concentration of DNA at pH=7 (DNA is in its natural hybridization state, forming a double chain) and at pH=12 (DNA has its chains mainly sepparated). The following graphs show the obtained results. D (density of DNA, in g·cm^{-3}, measured in a cesium chloride gradient) is represented in the X-axis. C (the relative concentration of DNA) is represented in the Y-axis. Observe the graphs and answer:

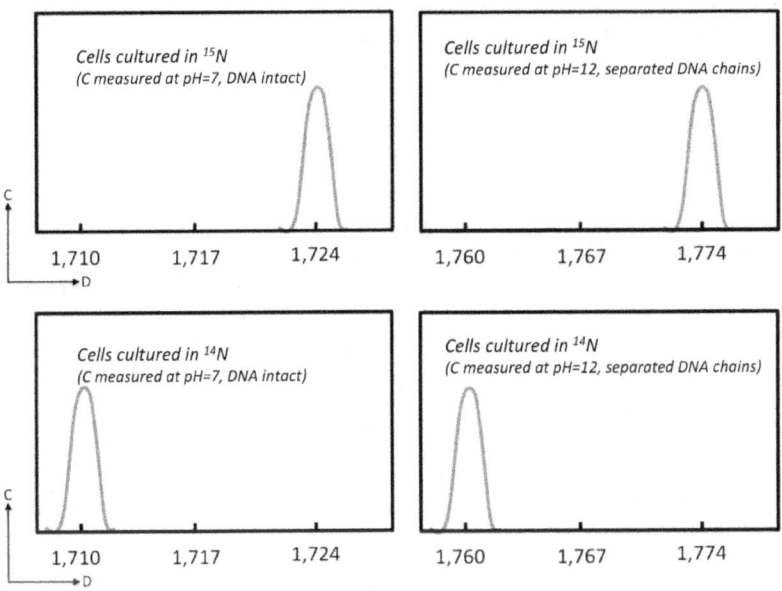

Imagine that cells are cultured with ^{15}N during one generation. Next, the medium is changed by other rich in ^{14}N. Finally, the relative concentration of DNA at pH=7 and pH=12 is measured. Which results will we obtain if DNA replication is semiconservative?

    a. at pH=7 we'll see an only peak at a density of 1.710 g·cm^{-3}
    b. at pH=12 we'll see an only peak at a density of 1.774 g·cm^{-3}
    c. at pH=7 we'll see an only peak at a density of 1.717 g·cm^{-3}
    d. at pH=12 we'll see an only peak at a density of 1.767 g·cm^{-3}
    e. at pH=7 we'll see two peaks, one at 1.710 and other at 1.717 g·cm^{-3}

473. Indicate which of the following assertions on secondary structure of DNA is true...

a. A and B forms are levorotary, and Z form is dextrorotary
b. the form with a largest number of base-pairs per helix turn is B form
c. the form with a largest linear length per helix turn is A form (~2.8 nm)
d. the A form is levorotary
e. the A form has approximately 11 base-pairs for each helix turn

474. B-DNA is more stable than A-DNA. In low humidity conditions, DNA prefers to be in A form. The physicochemical explanation for this behaviour is as follows:

a. in the major groove of B form, a column of water molecules (spine of hydration) can be formed, thus stabilizing B form
b. the flexibility of A form is greater and is entropically favoured in absence of solvent
c. the sum of individual interactions of water molecules with the phosphate groups of DNA in B form is less favourable than in the case of A form
d. A form, since it is levorotary, displays phosphate groups in a way that, in absence of water, diminishes electrostatic repulsion if compared to B form
e. A form can be more easily separated (both chains are deshybridized) than B form. So, A form is more favourable when it comes to entropy. In presence of water, the entropy generated by the movement of solvent molecules contributes much more to free energy than the tendency of the chains of DNA to be separated, thus masking the preference of DNA towards A form.

475. Indicate which of the following assertions on the main forms of DNA secondary structure (A, B and Z) is true...

a. the width of major and minor grooves is clearly different in B form
b. the width of major and minor grooves is almost identical in A form
c. looking at 3D structure of A and B forms from a point of view transversal to 5'→3' direction, A form has a central 'hole' and B form does not have it
d. only a and b are right
e. all the previous assertions are true

476. Within cells, the majority of DNA helices are supercoiled (that is, forming helicoidal structures of a higher level to that of double helix). When it comes to this, indicate which is the true option:

a. if the superhelix is levorotary, we say that supercoiling is positive, and if it is dextrorotary we say that supercoiling is negative
b. if the superhelix is levorotary, we say that supercoiling is negative, and if it is dextrorotary we say that supercoiling is positive
c. dextrorotary superhelices have not been observed in living cells extracts
d. levorotary superhelices have not been observed in living cells extracts
e. the change in turn sign of a superhelix, for the same DNA fragment, is so frequent that scientists accept to omit the nomenclature +/- for its description

477. DNA gyrase of E. coli...

a. introduces into DNA superhelicoidal levorotary turns
b. introduces into DNA superhelicoidal dextrorotary turns
c. uses ATP hydrolysis as energy source
d. a and c are right
e. b and c are right

478. A DNA topoisomerase is an enzyme that...

a. releases mechanical tension from supercoiled DNA fibers
b. allows DNA fluctuation among several topoisomers
c. cut and paste again supercoiled DNAs, thus releasing the mechanical tension that they accumulate
d. a and b are right
e. a, b and c are right

479. C-type DNA is a secondary structure obtained after submitting this polymer to high concentrations of Li$^+$ cation. An helix turn of this structure has 9.3 basepairs. It's...

a. ...an structure more coiled (less basepairs per turn) than the canonical B-type
b. ...an structure less coiled (more basepairs per turn) than the canonical B-type
c. ...a DNA with a larger interphosphate distance than the canonical B-type
d. a and c are right
e. b and c are right

480. Observe the following sequence of single chain DNA in which sub-sequences A, B, C, D and E have been indicated.

$^{5'}$ ACGCGTTTTTGAGACTCCCTAACCGATTCATGAATCCCCC $^{3'}$

A   B   C   D   E

Two sub-sequences are palindromic sequences. Which are they?

   a. B and E
   b. A and B
   c. A and D
   d. C and D
   e. A and C

481. Below, the sequence of 5'→3' chain of a series of DNA duplexes is written. Indicate which of them will presumably have the highest melting temperature (T_m)

A → ATATATATATATAT
B → TACGGATATATATA
C → TATATATACGCGCG
D → CGCGCGCGCGCGCG
E → CCCCCCCAAAAAAA

   a. A
   b. B
   c. C
   d. D
   e. E

482. After isolating the genetic material of a type of virus, its nucleotidic composition is analysed obtaining the following percentages. A=34%, C=11%, G=25%, T=30%. With this data we know that this genetic material is...

   a. double chain RNA
   b. single chain RNA
   c. double chain DNA
   d. single chain DNA
   e. a polypeptide of at least 100 100 amino acids

483. Some cell cultures grow in presence of several isotopes of nitrogen (^{15}N or ^{14}N). Next we measure the relative concentration of DNA at pH=7 (DNA is in its natural hybridization state, forming a double chain) and at pH=12 (DNA has its chains mainly sepparated). The following graphs show the obtained results. D (density of DNA, in g·cm^{-3}, measured in a cesium chloride gradient) is represented in the X-axis. C (the relative concentration of DNA) is represented in the Y-axis. Observe the graphs and answer:

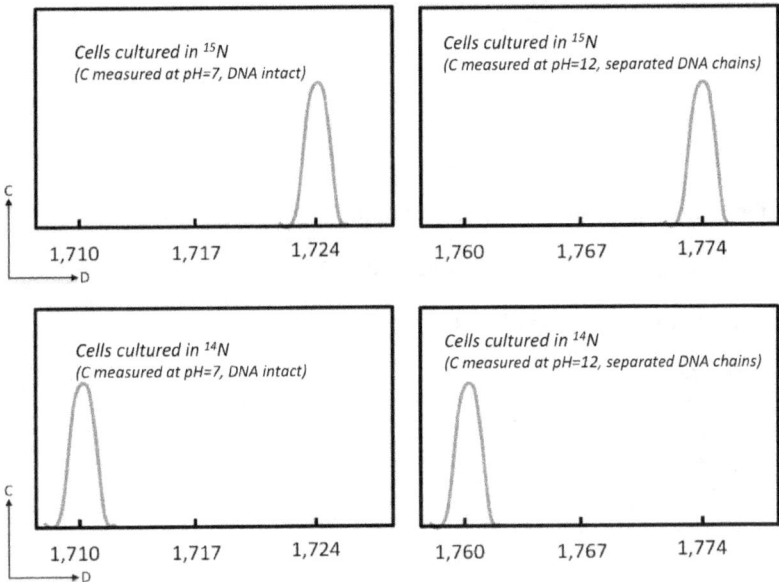

Imagine that cells are cultured with ^{15}N during one generation. Next, the medium is changed by other rich in ^{14}N and this medium is maintained during two more generations. Finally, the relative concentration of DNA at pH=7 and pH=12 is measured. Which results will we obtain if DNA replication is semiconservative?

a. at pH=7 we'll see an only peak at a density of 1.710 g·cm^{-3}
b. at pH=12 we'll see an only peak at a density of 1.774 g·cm^{-3}
c. at pH=7 we'll see an only peak at a density of 1.717 g·cm^{-3}
d. at pH=12 we'll see a small peak at a density of 1.760 g·cm^{-3} and a much higher peak at a density of 1.774 g·cm^{-3}
e. at pH=7 we'll see two peaks of almost the same height, one at 1.710 and other at 1.717 g·cm^{-3}

484. Below, the sequence of 5'→3' chain of a series of DNA duplexes is written. Indicate which of them will presumably have the lowest melting temperature (T$_m$)

A → ATATATATATATAT

B → TACGGATATATATA

C → TATATATACGCGCG

D → CGCGCGCGCGCGCG

E → CCCCCCCAAAAAAA

    a. A
    b. B
    c. C
    d. D
    e. E

485. Given the following sequence, corresponding to a double chain DNA,...

5' ATCTCTACTCAGG 3'

...write the complementary chain of DNA.

    a. 5' CCTGAGTAGAGAT 3'
    b. 5' CCUGWATERGAGAU 3'
    c. 3' CCTGAGTAGAGAT 5'
    d. 3' CCUGWATERGAGAU 5'
    e. 5' TAGAGATGAGTCC 3'

486. Given the following sequence, corresponding to a double chain DNA,...

5' ATCTCTACTCAGG 3'

...write the complementary chain of RNA coming from the transcription of the shown chain.

    a. 5' CCTGAGTAGAGAT 3'
    b. 5' CCUGWATERGAGAU 3'
    c. 3' CCTGAGTAGAGAT 5'
    d. 3' CCUGWATERGAGAU 5'
    e. 5' TAGAGATGAGTCC 3'

Bioenergetics and introduction to metabolism

487. This is a simplified and general schema of catabolism in an eukaryote cell. Indicate which molecules are represented by the A, B, C and D compounds?

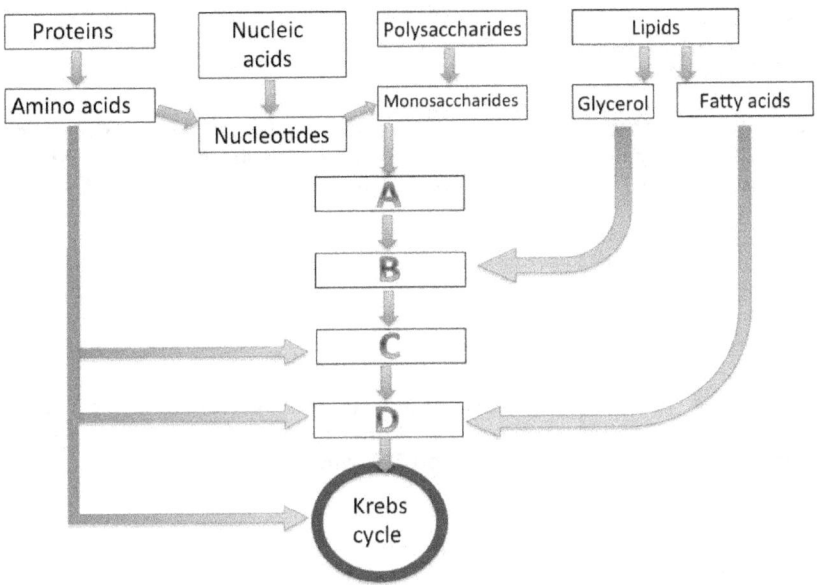

a. fructose-1.6-bisP / malate / CO_2 / lactate
b. glucose / fructose-1.6-bisP / lactate / CO_2
c. glycogen / fructose-1.6-bisP / pyruvate / glyceraldehyde-3-P
d. glycogen / fructose-1.6-bisP / $NADH+H^+$ / acetylCoA
e. glucose / glyceraldehyde-3-P / pyruvate / acetylCoA

488. The enzyme phosphoglucomutase catalyzes the transformation of glucose-1-phosphate into glucose-6-phosphate. At pH=7 and temperature=25°C, the K'_{eq} for this reaction is 19, what is its $\Delta G'^\circ$?

a. -0.08 kJ/mol
b. -3.17 kJ/mol
c. -7.30 kJ/mol
d. -82.16 kJ/mol
e. -7295.94 kJ/mol

489. The enzyme aspartate aminotransferase catalyzes the transformation of glutamate and oxaloacetate en aspartate and α-ketoglutarate. A pH=7 and temperature=25°C, la K'$_{eq}$ de esta reacción es de 6,8, ¿cuál es su $\Delta G'^o$?

a. -0,05 kJ/mol
b. -2,06 kJ/mol
c. -4,74 kJ/mol
d. -53,49 kJ/mol
e. -4749,89 kJ/mol

490. La enzyme triosa phosphate isomerase catalyzes the transformation of Dihydroxyacetone phosphate en glyceraldehyde-3-phosphate. A pH=7 and temperature=25°C, la K'$_{eq}$ de esta reacción es de 0,0475, ¿cuál es su $\Delta G'^o$?

a. 0,09 kJ/mol
b. 3,28 kJ/mol
c. 7,55 kJ/mol
d. 85,02 kJ/mol
e. 7550,13 kJ/mol

491. La enzyme phosphofructokinase catalyzes the transformation of fructose-6-phosphate and ATP into fructose-1,6-bisphosphate and ADP. At pH=7 and temperature=25°C, the K'$_{eq}$ for this reaction 254, what's its $\Delta G'^o$?

a. -0.15 kJ/mol
b. -5.96 kJ/mol
c. -13.72 kJ/mol
d. -154.51 kJ/mol
e. -13720.79 kJ/mol

492. Dissociation of acetic acid...

$$CH_3COOH + H_2O \rightarrow CH_3COO^- + H_3O^+$$

...has a constant K_a = 1,75x10-5. Calculate ΔG of this reaction at pH=0.

a. -13.10 kcal/mol
b. -1.31 kcal/mol
c. 1.31 kcal/mol
d. 6.49 kcal/mol
e. 13.3 kcal/mol

493. Which of the writen formulas is right in relation to the following chemical reaction?

$$aA + bB \longrightarrow cC + dD$$

A $\Delta G = \Delta G'^\circ + RT \ln ([C]^c[D]^d/[A]^a[B]^b)$

B $\Delta G'^\circ = \Delta G + RT \ln ([C]^c[D]^d/[A]^a[B]^b)$

C $\Delta G = -RT \ln ([C]^c[D]^d/[A]^a[B]^b)$

D $\Delta G = \Delta G'^\circ + RT \ln ([A]^a[B]^b/[C]^c[D]^d)$

E $0 = \Delta G - RT \ln ([A]^a[B]^b/[C]^c[D]^d)$

a. A
b. B
c. C
d. D
e. E

494. The enzyme phosphoglucomutase catalyzes the transformation of glucose-1-phosphate into glucose-6-phosphate. The K'_{eq} of this reaction at pH=7 and temperature=25°C is 19, which are the concentrations of glucose-1-phosphate and glucose-6-phosphate at equilibrium?

a. [glucose-1-phosphate]=1mM ; [glucose-6-phosphate]=19mM
b. [glucose-1-phosphate]=19mM ; [glucose-6-phosphate]=1mM
c. [glucose-1-phosphate]=18mM ; [glucose-6-phosphate]=1mM
d. [glucose-1-phosphate]=1mM ; [glucose-6-phosphate]=20mM
e. [glucose-1-phosphate]=20mM ; [glucose-6-phosphate]=18mM

495. $\Delta G'^\circ$ for ATP hydrolysis, as expressed by the following reaction, is -30.5 kJ/mol. If the concentrations of ATP, ADP and P_i, within human erythrocytes, are 2.25 mM, 0.25 mM and 1.65 mM, respectively, pH is 7.0 and temperature is 37°C. Which is the value of ΔG in these conditions?

$$ATP \longrightarrow ADP + P_i$$

a. -8.32 kJ/mol
b. -22.18 kJ/mol
c. -39.10 kJ/mol
d. -52.68 kJ/mol
e. -22209.13 J/mol

179

496. $\Delta G'^o$ for glutamine hydrolysis, to form glutamate and NH4+ is -11.4 kJ/mol. If the concentrations of glutamine, glutamate and NH4+, within human hepatocytes, are 0.6 mM, 0.05 mM and 0.2 M, respectively, pH is 7.0 and temperature is 37°C. Which is ΔG in these conditions?

a. -0.85 kJ/mol
b. −10.55 kJ/mol
c. -15.49 kJ/mol
d. -10565.19 J/mol
e. -21953.79 J/mol

497. Chemical reactions causing bioluminiscence in fireflies are the following:

a. Luciferase enzyme takes luciferyl adenylate, combines it with O_2 and forms oxyluciferin. In this reaction CO_2, AMP and visible light are released. Oxyluciferin, through a series of reactions, generates luciferin, that by addition of AMP, regenerates luciferyl adenylate, closing the cycle.
b. Luciferase enzyme takes luciferyl adenylate, combines it with O_2 and forms oxyluciferin. In this reaction CO_2, AMP and visible light are released. Oxyluciferin, by addition of AMP, is transformed again into luciferin, closing the cycle.
c. Luciferin deshydrogenase enzyme takes luciferyl adenylate, combines it with O_2 and forms oxyluciferin. In this reaction CO_2, AMP and visible light are released. Oxyluciferin, by addition of AMP, is transformed again into luciferin, closing the cycle.
d. Oxyluciferin transforms into luciferin, by luciferin oxidase enzyme, in a reaction in which O_2, ATP and visible light are released. Luciferin, in a short time, is oxydized again into oxyluciferin, and the cycle is closed.
e. Oxyluciferin transforms into luciferin, by luciferin oxidase enzyme, in a reaction in which CO_2, AMP and visible light are released. Luciferin, in a short time, is oxydized again into oxyluciferin, and the cycle is closed.

498. Which of the following assertions is FALSE?

a. NADH presents an absorbance maximum ata wavelength of 260 nm.
b. NAD+ presents an absorbance maximum at a wavelength of 260 nm and other maximum, with lower intensity, at ~340 nm.
c. NADH acts as an electron transporter in soluble form.
d. NADH is composed by two nucleotides bound by their phosphate groups.
e. The nicotinamide ring is plain in NAD+ and loses planarity in NADH.

499. NADH and NADPH coenzymes have a purine base that is adenine, and a pyrimidine base that is...

a. Thymine
b. Nicotinamide
c. Nicotindiamide
d. Cytidinamide
e. Nystatin

500. We add a catalytic amount of glucose-6-phosphatase to a water solution of glucose-6-phosphate. When equilibrium is reached, the concentration of glucose-6-phosphate is 0.5 mM, of glucose is 0.2 M and of inorganic phosphate (P$_i$) is 0.53 M. Knowing that the reaction is at pH = 7, temperature = 37°C, which is $\Delta G'^\circ$ for this reaction?

a. -13807 kJ/mol
b. -15.44 kJ/mol
c. −13.81 kJ/mol
d. 13.81 kJ/mol
e. 15.44 kJ/mol

501. ATP hydrolysis...

a. decreases the acidity of the medium
b. increases the acidity of the medium
c. does not affect to pH of the medium
d. only affects to pH if it's coupled to the phosphorylation of a protein
e. only affects to pH if it's coupled to the formation of NADH + H⁺

502. $\Delta G'^\circ$ for ATP hydrolysis...

a. becomes more positive as the pH of the medium increases
b. becomes more negative as the pH of the medium increases
c. varies exponentially as the pH of the medium changes in a linear way
d. a and c are right
e. b and c are right

503. $\Delta G'^{o}$ for ATP hydrolysis...

a. varies in the range between -7 kcal/mol and -9 kcal/mol as [Mg^{2+}] varies in the range from 0 to 50 mM
b. at almost null concentrations of Mg^{2+}, is lower than -8 kcal/mol, later it rises until approximately -7 kcal/mol and becomes more negative as the pH of the medium increases
c. varies exponentially as the pH of the medium changes in a linear way
d. a and c are right
e. b and c are right

504. Which of the following assertions in relation to ATP hydrolysis are right?

$$ATP \rightarrow ADP + P_i$$

A → entropy of products is higher than entropy of reactives
B → ΔG of solvation for the products is more negative than for the reactives
C → products are better stabilized by resonance than reactives
D → electrostatic repulsion (mainly between phosphates) has lower intensity in products than in reactives

a. only A and D
b. only B and D
c. only B, C and D
d. only A, B and C
e. A, B, C and D

505. NADH and NADPH coenzymes have a purine base and a pyrimidine base. The purine base is adenine, the pyrimidine base is nicotinamide...

a. ...and it's formed by decarboxylation of thymine
b. ...and it's formed from niacid, that is made from tryptophan
c. ...and it's made from nicotinic acid, that is made by nicotine transaminase from α-cetoglutarate and glutamine
d. ... and it is made from coenzyme B_{12}
e. ... and it's made from nicotinic acid, that is made by nicotine transaminase from α-ketoglutarate and thymine

506. Aldolase catalyzes the following reaction within glycolysis...

Fructose-1,6-bisP → Dihydroxyacetone-P + Glyceraldehyde-3-P

...that we can write in a simplified form as FbP→DHP+G3P.

Knowing that $\Delta G^{0'}$ for this reaction is 5.5 kcal mol^{-1} (pH=7; 25°C). Calculate [G3P] at equilibrium if the initial concentration of FbP is 1 M.

  a. 9.5 M
  b. 0.95 M
  c. 0.095 M
  d. 0.0095 M
  e. 0.00095 M

507. Experiment A.

ATP with the phosphate γ radioactively labelled with ^{32}P is added to a yeast extract. An hour later, the soluble fraction, corresponding to P_i is isolated and the amount of $^{32}P_i$ radioactive found ddddis measured.

Experiment B.

ATP with the phosphate β radioactively labelled with ^{32}P is added to a yeast extract. An hour later, the soluble fraction, corresponding to P_i is isolated and the amount of $^{32}P_i$ radioactive found ddddis measured.

Which behaviour will be most likely derived from results?

  a. in experiment A we find more ^{32}P in the P_i fraction than in experiment B
  b. in experiment B we find more ^{32}P in the P_i fraction than in experiment A
  c. in both experiments A and B we find moreless the same amount of ^{32}P in the P_i fraction, that will be presumably elevated due to the high consumption of ATP made by yeast
  d. in both experiments A and B we find moreless the same amount of ^{32}P in the P_i fraction, that will be almost zero since yeast scarcely consume ATP
  e. in both experiments A and B we find moreless the same amount of ^{32}P in the P_i fraction, that will be almost zero since radioactivity is rapidly lost after ATP hydrolysis

508. The following reaction...

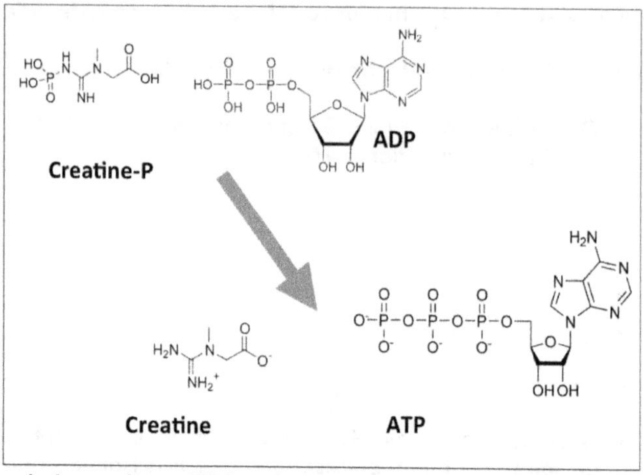

...occurs at muscle to produce ATP in a fast manner. The concentrations of reactives and products when this reaction reaches equilibrium are as follows:

[creatineP] = 25 mM
[ADP] = 0,013mM
[creatine] = 13 mM
[ATP] = 4 mM

$\Delta G'^o$ for ATP hydrolysis is –7.3 kcal/mol. Calculate $\Delta G'^o$ for the hydrolysis of creatine-P.

Creatine-P + H_2O → Creatine + P_i

a. -9.5 kcal/mol
b. -10.3 kcal/mol
c. -11.1 kcal/mol
d. -46.40 kJ/mol
e. c and d are right

509. Many metabolic processes are activated or inhibited in response to the relative concentrations of adenine nucleotides. The concentrations of AMP, ADP and ATP within a cell are indicative of the rate of certain pathways, such as glycolysis. Atkinson propused, to measure this state of the cell, a parameter named "adenylate energy charge" How is this parameter calculated?

    a. ([ATP]+([ADP]/2)) / ([ATP]+[ADP]+[AMP])
    b. ([ADP]+[ATP]) / ([ATP]+[ADP]+[AMP])
    c. ([ATP]+[ADP]) / ([ATP]+[AMP])
    d. ([ATP]+([ADP]/2)) / (([ATP]/2)+[ADP]+([AMP]/2))
    e. ([ADP]+([AMP]/2)) / ([ATP]+[ADP]+[AMP])

510. If adding adequate amounts of the enzyme glucose-6-phosphatase to a 0.1 M solution of glucose-6-P, when the reaction of phosphate release...

$$glucose\text{-}6\text{-}phosphate + H_2O \rightarrow Glucose + P_i$$

...reaches equilibrium, the amount of glucose-6-phosphate has been reduced until being only 0.05% of its initial value. Calculate $\Delta G'^o$ for the synthesis of glucosa-6-phosphate (the reverse reaction to that shown above). Other conditions (pH=7; 25°C)

    a. 3.2 kcal/mol
    b. 4.0 kcal/mol
    c. -3200 cal/mol
    d. -4000 cal/mol
    e. 4.8 kcal/mol

511. The reaction of acetic acid dissociation...

$$CH_3COOH + H_2O \rightarrow CH_3COO^- + H_3O^+$$

...has a constant $K_a = 1{,}75 \times 10^{-5}$. Calculate ΔG of this reaction at pH=5.

    a. -13.10 kcal/mol
    b. -1.31 kcal/mol
    c. 1.31 kcal/mol
    d. 6.49 kcal/mol
    e. 13.3 kcal/mol

512. Calculate ΔG of ATP hydrolysis in the following conditions. pH=7; T=25°C; [ATP]=10^{-3}M; [ADP]=10^{-4}M; [P_i]=10^{-2}M; $\Delta G'^0$ (pH=7, 25°C) = -7.7 kcal mol^{-1}

a. -11.79 kcal/mol
b. -7.70 kcal/mol
c. -3.96 kcal/mol
d. 2.55 kcal/mol
e. 16.62 kcal/mol

513. Calculate K'eq of glucose phosphorylation by hexokinase...

$$\text{Glucose + ATP} \rightarrow \text{Glucose-6-P + ADP}$$

...knowing that $\Delta G'^0$ for ATP hydrolysis is -7.7 kcal.mol^{-1} and $\Delta G'^0$ of glucose-6-P hydrolysis is -3.14 kcal mol^{-1} (both reactions at 25°C and pH = 7)

a. $-8.21 \cdot 10^3$
b. $-5.21 \cdot 10^3$
c. $2.21 \cdot 10^3$
d. $5.21 \cdot 10^3$
e. $8.21 \cdot 10^3$

514. Aldolase catalyzes the following reaction within glycolysis...

$$\text{Fructose-1,6-bisP} \rightarrow \text{Dihydroxyacetone-P + Glyceraldehyde-3-P}$$

...that can be written in a simpler way as FbP$\rightarrow$DHP+G3P.

Knowing that $\Delta G^{0'}$ for this reaction is 5.5 kcal mol^{-1} (pH=7; 25°C). Calculate [G3P] at equilibrium if the initial concentration of FbP is 0.01 M.

a. 9.5 M
b. 0.95 M
c. 0.095 M
d. 0.0095 M
e. 0.00095 M

Sugar metabolism

Absortion and transport of sugars

515. Intestinal maltase catalyzes the following reaction...
   a. maltose → 2 D-glucose
   b. maltose + H_2O → 2 D-glucose
   c. maltose → D-glucose + D-fructose
   d. maltose + H_2O → D-glucose + D-fructose
   e. maltose + H_2O → D-glucose + D-mannose

516. Hexoses dissolved in the intestinal liquid pass to the liver through...
   a. saphenous vein
   b. aorta artery
   c. ulnar vein
   d. cystic artery
   e. hepatic portal vein

517. How is the glucose absorbed at an intestinal level?
   a. By an antiport transport coupled to Na^+ recruitment.
   b. By a symport transport coupled to Na^+ recruitment.
   c. By an antiport transport coupled to K^+ recruitment.
   d. By a symport transport coupled to K^+ recruitment.
   e. By means of glucose channels named GLUT, of which there are several described types (GLUT1, GLUT2, GLUT3 and GLUT4)

518. Intestinal sucrase catalyzes the following reaction...
   a. sucrose + H_2O → 2 D-glucose
   b. sucrose + H_2O → D-glucose + D-galactose
   c. sucrose + H_2O → D-glucose + D-fructose
   d. sucrose + H_2O → L-glucose + D-galactose
   e. sucrose + H_2O → D-glucose + L-galactose

519. Intestinal lactase catalyzes the following reaction...
   a. sucrose + H_2O → 2 D-glucose
   b. sucrose + H_2O → D-glucose + D-galactose
   c. sucrose + H_2O → D-glucose + D-fructose
   d. sucrose + H_2O → L-glucose + D-galactose
   e. sucrose + H_2O → D-glucose + L-galactose

Glycolysis

520. Which option does contain the proper terms to fill the gaps in this fragment:

"Glycolysis is the transformation of a molecule of glucose, that has ____ carbon atoms, into 2 molecules of _____, each one with ____ carbon atoms. This process yields a net gain of ___ ATPs and ____ reduced coenzymes of the type ____. "

    a. 12, phosphoenolpyruvate, 6, 2, 2, NADH+H$^+$
    b. 6, pyruvate, 3, 2, 2, NADH+H$^+$
    c. 4, dihydroxyacetonephosphate, 2, 2, 2, NADH+H$^+$
    d. 6, pyruvate, 3, 2, 1, FADH$_2$
    e. 6, pyruvate, 3, 2, 1, NADH+H$^+$

521. Which of the following assertions is FALSE?

    a. glycolysis rate in a living tissue decreases in presence of O_2, what is know as 'Pasteur's effect'
    b. if a glycolysis active tissue is exposed to a high O_2 concentration, an increase in fructose-1,6-bisP concentration is observed, while the concentration of other glycolytic intermediates like fructose-6-P is reduced
    c. glycolysis rate depends on adenylate energy charge. When the charge is high, the pathway is inactive, and when it's low, the pathway activates
    d. AMP, ADP and fructose-2,6-bisP activate phosphofructokinase enzyme, and so the glycolytic pathway
    e. glycolysis rate grows as ATP concentration in the tissue decreases

522. Four glycolysis intermediates are molecules that normally adopt a cyclic form in aqueous solution. Which are?

    a. glyceraldehyde-3-P / galactose-1-P / glucose / dihydroxyacetone-P
    b. phosphoenolpyruvate / glucose / 2-phosphoglycerate / 3-phosphoglycerate
    c. fructose-1,6-bisP / fructose-2,6-bisP / pyruvate / phosphoenolpyruvate
    d. glucose-6-P / fructose-6-P / 1,3-bisPglycerate / phosphoenolpyruvate
    e. fructose-1,6-bisP / glucose / glucose-6-P / fructose-6-P

523. Glycolysis is the transformation of glucose into pyruvate, through the following sequence of compounds, in the order indicated below:

a. glucose → glucose-6-phosphate → fructose-6-phosphate → fructose-1,6-bisphosphate → (dihydroxyacetone-phosphate + glyceraldehyde-3-phosphate) → 1,3-bisphosphoglycerate → 3-phosphoglycerate → 2-phosphoglycerate → phosphoenolpyruvate → pyruvate

b. glucose → fructose-6-phosphate → fructose-1,6-bisphosphate → glyceraldehyde-3-phosphate → 1,3-bisphosphoglycerate → 3-phosphoglycerate → phosphoenolpyruvate → pyruvate

c. glucose → glucose-6-phosphate → fructose-6-phosphate → (dihydroxyacetone-phosphate + glyceraldehyde-3-phosphate) → 1,3-bisphosphoglycerate → 3-phosphoglycerate → phosphoenolpyruvate → pyruvate

d. glucose → glucose-6-phosphate → fructose-1,6-bisphosphate → (dihydroxyacetone-phosphate + glyceraldehyde-3-phosphate) → 1,3-bisphosphoglycerate → 3-phosphoglycerate → 2-phosphoglycerate → phosphoenolpyruvate → pyruvate

e. glucose → glucose-6-phosphate → glucose-1,6-bisphosphate → (dihydroxyacetone-phosphate + glyceraldehyde-3-phosphate) → 1,3-bisphosphoglycerate → 3-phosphoglycerate → 2-phosphoglycerate → phosphoenolpyruvate → pyruvate

524. Glycolysis is the transformation of glucose into pyruvate, through the following sequence of compounds, in the order indicated below. Each compound has a number of carbon atoms (specified within brakets). Which is the right option?

a. glucose (6) → glucose-6-phosphate (6) → fructose-6-phosphate (6) → fructose-1,6-bisphosphate (6) → (dihydroxyacetone-phosphate (4) + glyceraldehyde-3-phosphate (2)) → 1,3-bisphosphoglycerate (3) → 3-phosphoglycerate (3) → 2-phosphoglycerate (3) → phosphoenolpyruvate (3) → pyruvate (3)

b. glucose (6) → glucose-6-phosphate (6) → fructose-6-phosphate (6) → fructose-1,6-bisphosphate (6) → (dihydroxyacetone-phosphate (2) + glyceraldehyde-3-phosphate (4)) → 1,3-bisphosphoglycerate (3) → 3-phosphoglycerate (3) → 2-phosphoglycerate (3) → phosphoenolpyruvate (3) → pyruvate (3)

c. glucose (6) → glucose-6-phosphate (6) → fructose-6-phosphate (6) → fructose-1,6-bisphosphate (6) → (dihydroxyacetone-phosphate (3) + glyceraldehyde-3-phosphate (3)) → 1,3-bisphosphoglycerate (3) → 3-phosphoglycerate (3) → 2-phosphoglycerate (2) → phosphoenolpyruvate (2) → pyruvate (2)

d. glucose (6) → glucose-6-phosphate (6) → fructose-6-phosphate (6) → fructose-1,6-bisphosphate (6) → (dihydroxyacetone-phosphate (2) + glyceraldehyde-3-phosphate (4)) → 1,3-bisphosphoglycerate (4) → 3-phosphoglycerate (4) → 2-phosphoglycerate (4) → phosphoenolpyruvate (3) → pyruvate (3)

e. glucose (6) → glucose-6-phosphate (6) → fructose-6-phosphate (6) → fructose-1,6-bisphosphate (6) → (dihydroxyacetone-phosphate (3) + glyceraldehyde-3-phosphate (3)) → 1,3-bisphosphoglycerate (3) → 3-phosphoglycerate (3) → 2-phosphoglycerate (3) → phosphoenolpyruvate (3) → pyruvate (3)

525. Which of the following assertions is FALSE?

a. ATP binds allosterically to phosphofructokinase, reducing its affinity for fructose-6-P and slowing glycolysis

b. Glucagon, through protein kinase A, inhibits phosphofructokinase-2, reducing [fructose-2,6-bisP], and thus inhibiting phosphofructokinase-1 activity

c. Citrate binds allosterically to phosphofructokinase, reducing its activity and slowing glycolysis

d. the allosteric and inhibitory action of ATP on phosphofructokinase-1 becomes more intense as pH increases

e. Phosphoenolpyruvate binds allosterically to phosphofructokinase, reducing its activity and slowing glycolysis

526. Glycolysis is the transformation of glucose into pyruvate, through the following sequence of compounds, in the order indicated below. Each compound has a number of oxygen atoms (specified within brakets). Which is the right option?

a. glucose (6) → glucose-6-phosphate (6) → fructose-6-phosphate (6) → fructose-1,6-bisphosphate (6) → (dihydroxyacetone-phosphate (3) + glyceraldehyde-3-phosphate (3)) → 1,3-bisphosphoglycerate (3) → 3-phosphoglycerate (3) → 2-phosphoglycerate (3) → phosphoenolpyruvate (3) → pyruvate (3)

b. glucose (6) → glucose-6-phosphate (6) → fructose-6-phosphate (6) → fructose-1,6-bisphosphate (6) → (dihydroxyacetone-phosphate (4) + glyceraldehyde-3-phosphate (5)) → 1,3-bisphosphoglycerate (6) → 3-phosphoglycerate (6) → 2-phosphoglycerate (6) → phosphoenolpyruvate (4) → pyruvate (4)

c. glucose (6) → glucose-6-phosphate (9) → fructose-6-phosphate (9) → fructose-1,6-bisphosphate (12) → (dihydroxyacetone-phosphate (6) + glyceraldehyde-3-phosphate (6)) → 1,3-bisphosphoglycerate (6) → 3-phosphoglycerate (6) → 2-phosphoglycerate (6) → phosphoenolpyruvate (6) → pyruvate (3)

d. glucose (6) → glucose-6-phosphate (9) → fructose-6-phosphate (9) → fructose-1,6-bisphosphate (12) → (dihydroxyacetone-phosphate (6) + glyceraldehyde-3-phosphate (6)) → 1,3-bisphosphoglycerate (10) → 3-phosphoglycerate (7) → 2-phosphoglycerate (7) → phosphoenolpyruvate (6) → pyruvate (3)

e. glucose (6) → glucose-6-phosphate (7) → fructose-6-phosphate (7) → fructose-1,6-bisphosphate (8) → (dihydroxyacetone-phosphate (4) + glyceraldehyde-3-phosphate (4)) → 1,3-bisphosphoglycerate (5) → 3-phosphoglycerate (4) → 2-phosphoglycerate (4) → phosphoenolpyruvate (4) → pyruvate (3)

527. The enzymes that transfer phosphate groups, like hexokinase or phosphofructokinase-1, need to have in the active site a cation for the proper behaviour of the catalytic mechanism. Which is this cation?

a. Na^+
b. K^+
c. Ca^{2+}
d. Mn^{2+}
e. Mg^{2+}

528. La phosphoglucose isomerase...

a. catalyzes the transformation of glucose-6-P into glucose-1-P
b. catalyzes the transformation of glucose-6-P into UDP-galactose
c. catalyzes the transformation of glucose-6-P into fructose-6-P
d. catalyzes the transformation of glucose-6-P into fructose-1,6-bisP
e. catalyzes the transformation of glucose-6-P into fructose-1-P

529. Which of the following assertions is FALSE?

a. Pyruvate kinasa is inhibited by high ATP concentrations
b. Fructose-1,6-bisP allosterically activates pyruvate kinase
c. AcetylCoA activates pyruvate kinase
d. a and c
e. b and c

530. La hexokinase...

a. catalyzes the transformation of glucose into glucose-1-P
b. catalyzes the transformation of glucose into UDP-galactose
c. catalyzes the transformation of glucose into fructose-6-P
d. catalyzes the transformation of glucose into fructose-1,6-bisP
e. catalyzes the transformation of glucose into glucose-6-P

531. Phosphofructokinase1...

a. catalyzes the transformation of glucose-6-P into glucose-1-P
b. catalyzes the transformation of fructose-6-P into fructose-1,6-bisP
c. catalyzes the transformation of glucose into fructose-6-P
d. catalyzes the transformation of glucose-6-P into fructose-1,6-bisP
e. catalyzes the transformation of glucose-6-P into fructose-6-P

532. Louis Pasteur observed a behaviour in the glycolytic pathway known today as 'Pasteur effect' What is it about?
   a. Glycolysis stopped in presence of strong acids
   b. While yeasts are degrading glucose, they are exposed to crescent concentrations of ethanol, thus deriving glycolytic pathway towards lactate production
   c. The rate of glycolytic pathway is higher in yeasts that are simultaneously feeded with fatty acids
   d. Adding ethanol to a yeast cell culture results in an accumulation of pyruvate and stops glycolytic pathway
   e. The rate of glycolysis drastically drops when the culture of yeasts is exposed to air

533. Phosphofructokinase2...
   a. catalyzes the transformation of glucose-6-P into fructose-2,6-bisP
   b. catalyzes the transformation of fructose-6-P into fructose-2,6-bisP
   c. catalyzes the transformation of fructose-1,6-bisP into fructose-2,6-bisP
   d. catalyzes the transformation of glucose into fructose-2,6-bisP
   e. catalyzes the change of fructose-1,6-bisP into fructose-2,6-bisP, and vice versa

534. In the human body, the transformation of glucose into glucose-6-P ...

   a. is catalysed by one of three existent types of hexokinases, it consumes 1 ATP molecule, and requires the presence of Ca^{2+} in the catalytic site
   b. is catalysed by one of four existent types of hexokinases, it consumes 2 ATP molecules, and requires the presence of Mg^{2+} in the catalytic site
   c. is catalysed by one of four existent types of hexokinases, it consumes 2 ATP molecules, and requires the presence of K^+ in the catalytic site
   d. is catalysed by one of three existent types of hexokinases, it consumes 2 ATP molecules, and requires the presence of K^+ in the catalytic site
   e. is catalysed by one of four existent types of hexokinases, it consumes 1 ATP molecule, and requires the presence of Mg^{2+} in the catalytic site

535. Which of the following assertions on sugar entrance to glycolysis is FALSE?

   a. Each galactose that enters glycolysis consumes previously 1 ATP to be transformed into galactose-1-P.
   b. Each galactose that enters glycolysis was iniatially in the form of galactose-1-P, then an UDP is transferred and it converts into UDP-galactose.
   c. UDP-galactose is transformed into UDP-glucose by glucose epimerase enzyme.
   d. UDP-glucose transfers UDP to galactose-1-P and becomes glucose-1-P. This is catalysed by the UDP-glucose-galactose-1-P uridylyltransferase enzyme.
   e. Phosphoglucomutase takes then glucose-1-P and converts it into fructose-6-P, changing the place of phosphate group and the position of anomeric carbon.

536. To which pathway does the following picture correspond?

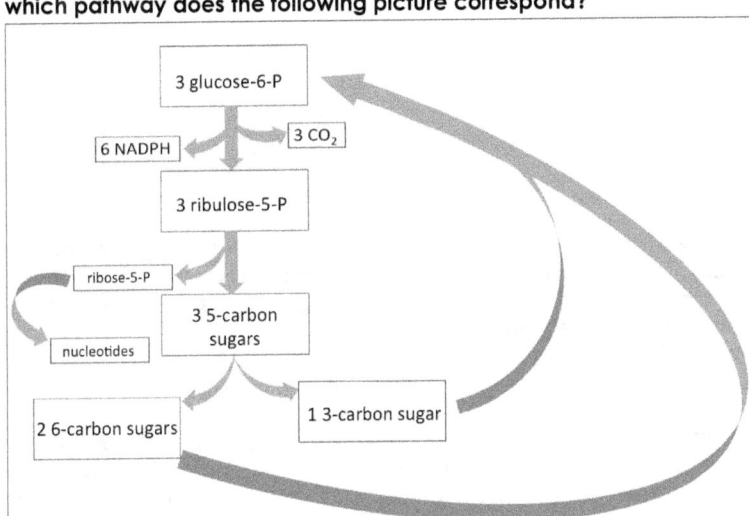

a. anaplerotic reactions associated to Krebs cycle
b. pentose phosphate pathway
c. Calvin cycle
d. Krebs cycle
e. glyoxylate cycle

537. In glycolysis, for each glucose, 2 molecules of NADH + 2H⁺ are generated. Specifically, which enzyme is in charge of this step?

a. hexokinase
b. pyruvate dehydrogenase
c. fructose bisphosphate aldolase
d. glyceraldehyde dehydrogenase
e. phosphoglyceratekinase

538. For glycolysis to have a net favourable energetic balance (in the form of 2 ATPs for each glucose that enters the pathway) it's needed a high energy phosphotriose to be generated in one of its steps, which enzyme is in charge of this step?

a. hexokinase
b. pyruvate dehydrogenase
c. fructose bisphosphate aldolase
d. glyceraldehyde dehydrogenase
e. phosphoglyceratekinase

539. Phosphofructokinase1 adds a phosphate group to its substrate, fructose-6-P, to which carbon is it attached?

a. 1
b. 2
c. 3
d. 4
e. 5

540. In most of body tissues, fructose enters glycolysis at the level of fructose-6-P. In hepatic cells, however, an slightly different pathway occurs. There, fructokinase phosphorilates carbon 1 of fructose generating fructose-1-P. Which is the most common use for this metabolite?

a. it's converted into fructose-6-P by hepatic fructose epimerase.
b. it's converted into fructose-1,6-bisP by hepatic phosphofructokinase.
c. it's decarboxylated and incorporated to pentose phosphate pathway.
d. it's broken by aldolase B, producing dihydroxyacetone-P and glyceraldehyde.
e. it's converted into glucose-1-P by an specific isomerase and then an epimerase transforms it into glucose-6-P.

541. Triose phosphate isomerase catalyzes the conversion of a triose with a _____ group into another with a _____ group.

a. enol / ketone
b. ketone / aldehyde
c. aldehyde / carboxyl
d. imino / amino
e. ketone / carboxyl

542. Phosphoglycerate mutase catalyzes the swap of a phosphate group among the carbons number ____ and ____ of phosphoglycerate.
a. 1 and 2
b. 1 and 3
c. 2 and 3
d. 1 and 4
e. 2 and 4

543. In the phosphoenolpyruvate to pyruvate transformation, pyruvate kinase consumes...
a. 1 ADP
b. 1 ADP + 1 NAD$^+$
c. 2 ADPs
d. 2 ADPs + 2 NAD$^+$
e. 2 NAD$^+$

544. 2-phosphoglycerate→phosphoenolpyruvate step, in enolase enzyme, entails...

a. the loss of 1 ATP
b. the gain of 1 ATP
c. the loss of an H_2O molecule
d. the loss of a CO_2 molecule
e. the loss of a phosphate group

545. 1,3-bisPglycerate→3-phosphoglycerate step, by phosphoglyceratekinase, entails...
a. the loss of 1 ATP
b. the gain of 1 ATP
c. the loss of an H_2O molecule
d. the loss of a CO_2 molecule
e. the loss of a phosphate group

546. The enzyme UDP-glucose pyrophosphorylase acts in glycolysis, which is its role?

a. To introduce heme group derivatives into the pathway
b. To prepare UDP-glucose, an activated precursor that will allow the entrance of galactose in the pathway
c. To transform glucose into fructose-1,6-bisP by an alternative pathway involving the formation of UDP-glucose and by-passing phosphofructokinase-1, hence escaping from classical regulation of glycolysis.
d. To break UDP-glucose producing fructose-1-P that, after the action of an epimerase, is transformed into fructose-6-P and enters the pathway.
e. To break fructose-6-P, generating inorganic phosphate (P_i) and producing an intermediate (UDP-glucose) that goes to pentose phosphate pathway. Fructose-1,6-bisP and citrate activate allosterically this enzyme, thus deviating the metabolic flux to other destinations when glycolysis rate is too high.

547. In the first phase of glycolysis, through 5 steps, glucose is transformed into 2 molecules of glyceraldehyde-3-P. Globally, when comparing a glucose (G) and 2 molecules of glyceraldehyde-3-P (G3P)...

a. the number of carbons and oxygens remains the same
b. the number of carbons and oxygens is halfway reduced, and a phosphorous appears in each G3P
c. the number of carbons is the same and the number of oxygens is duplicated
d. 1 atom of phosphorous, that was absent in G, appears in each G3P
e. c and d are right

548. The intermediates that appear at several steps of the transformation of glyceraldehyde-3-phosphate into pyruvate have one, zero or several phosphate groups. Including pyruvate and glyceraldehyde-3-P, if we write a series indicating only the number of phosphates for each compound, it would be as follows...

a. $1 \to 1 \to 2 \to 1 \to 1 \to 0$
b. $1 \to 1 \to 1 \to 1 \to 2 \to 1$
c. $1 \to 0 \to 1 \to 0 \to 0 \to 0$
d. $1 \to 2 \to 1 \to 1 \to 1 \to 0$
e. $1 \to 2 \to 2 \to 2 \to 1 \to 0$

549. Which two enzymes of glycolysis do consume ATP?
a. triose phosphate isomerase and glyceraldehydephosphate dehydrogenase
b. enolase and phosphoglycerate mutase
c. enolase and phosphofructokinase1
d. hexokinase and phosphofructokinase1
e. phosphoglycerate kinase and phosphoglucose isomerase

550. Ingested sucrose easily is transformed to fat by a pathway alternative to glycolysis that is specially active in the liver. This pathway allows to escape from the control of phosphofructokinase, which is this pathway?

a. fructose → fructose-1-P → dihydroxyacetone-P + glyceraldehyde → glycerol-3-P → triglycerides
b. fructose → fructose-1-P → fructose-6-P → fructose-1,6-bisP → dihydroxyacetone + glyceraldehyde-3-P → glycerol-3-P → triglycerides
c. glucose → glucose-1-P → pyruvate → glycerol-3-P → triglycerides
d. glucose + fructose → fructose-6-P → dihydroxyacetone + glyceraldehyde-3-P → glycerol-3-P → triglycerides
e. fructose → fructose-1,6-bisP → dihydroxyacetone-P + glyceraldehyde-3-P → glycerol-3-P → triglycerides

551. A reaction in glycolysis involves decarboxylation of substrate. It's catalysed by...

a. triose phosphate isomerase
b. enolase
c. phosphofructokinase1
d. hexokinase
e. none

Anaerobic fermentations of pyruvate

552. How many NADH+H⁺ molecules are produced by the oxidation of a molecule of glucose to two molecules of lactate?

    a. None. 2 are consumed, so the net balance is -2
    b. 0
    c. 1
    d. 2
    e. 4

553. In a type of alcoholic fermentation, pyruvate is transformed into ethanol. Which of the following assertions related to this process is FALSE?

    a. A NAD^+ molecule is reduced for each pyruvate molecule transformed
    b. It's a 2-step reaction that passes through acetaldehyde
    c. A CO_2 molecule is lost for each transformed pyruvate molecule
    d. The enzyme pyruvate decarboxylase participates in the process
    e. The enzyme alcohol dehydrogenase participates in the process

554. Which of these reactions does correspond to the transformation of glucose that occurs in lactic fermentation?

A. Glucose + $2NAD^+$ + 2 ADP + 2 P_i → 2 Lactate+ 2 NADH + 2 H^+ + 2 ATP + 2 H_2O

B. Glucose + 2 ATP + → 2 Lactate+ 2 ADP + 2 P_i + 2 H_2O

C. Glucose + 2 ADP + 2 P_i → 2 Lactate + 2 ATP + 2 H_2O

D. Glucose → 2 Lactate + 2 H_2O

E. Glucose + 3 ADP + 3 P_i → 3 Lactate + 3 ATP + 3 H_2O

---

    a. A
    b. B
    c. C
    d. D
    e. E

555. Pyruvate carboxylase, to transform pyruvate into acetaldehyde, needs a coenzyme named...

a. coenzyme A
b. NAD^+
c. riboflavin
d. niacin
e. thiamine pyrophosphate

556. If we could follow the path of every carbon atom of a glucose, by labelling it with ^{14}C, during its whole transformation to ethanol through the processes of glycolysis and alcoholic fermentation. Which carbons would appear finally in CO_2?

a. 1 and 2
b. 3 and 4
c. 5 and 6
d. 1 and 6
e. 2 and 5

557. How does glycerol, produced in fatty acids catabolism, mainly enter glycolysis?

a. It's oxidized to dihydroxyacetone by glycerol dehydrogenase. Later, the enzyme dihydroxyacetone-P kinase transforms it into dihydroxyacetone-P
b. It's phosphorylated by glycerol kinase and is transformed into glycerol-3-P. Later, glycerol-3-P dehydrogenase transforms it into dihydroxyacetone-P
c. The enzyme glycerol carboxykinase transforms it into lactate, producing the lost of a CO_2
d. The enzyme glycerol carboxykinase transforms it into malate, producing the lost of a CO_2
e. It's bound to another glycerol, by glycerol polymerase, forming glucose. Later, hexokinase converts it into glucose-6-P

558. If we could follow the path of every carbon atom of a glucose, by labelling it with ^{14}C, during its whole transformation to ethanol through the processes of glycolysis and alcoholic fermentation. Which carbons would end in ethanol?

a. 1, 2, 3 and 4
b. 3, 4, 5 and 6
c. 1, 3, 5 and 6
d. 1, 2, 5 and 6
e. 2, 3, 4 and 5

559. Which of the following assertions on lactate dehydrogenase is FALSE?

a. It is a tetrameric protein

b. The isoforms present in liver and heart are richer in M subunit than the ones found in skeletal striated muscle

c. The five existing isoenzymes are made by combinations of M and H subunits, giving rise to 5 distinct isoforms: H_4, MH_3, M_2H_2, M_3H and M_4.

d. A blood test revealing a high content of H_4 and MH_3 isoforms can be indicative of the destruction of cardiac tissue, as a consequence for example of a myocardial infarction

e. M and H subunits are different in their amino acid sequences

560. Which of these reactions does correspond to the transformation of glucose that occurs in alcoholic fermentation?

A. Glucose + 2 H^+ + 2 ADP + 2 P_i → 2 Ethanol + 2 CO_2 + 2 ATP + 2 H_2O

B. Glucose + 2 ATP + → 2 Ethanol + 2 ADP + 2 P_i + 2 H_2O

C. Glucose + 2 ADP + 2 P_i → 2 Ethanol + 2 ATP + 2 H_2O + 2 CO_2

D. Glucose + 2 NAD^+ + 2 ADP + 2 P_i → 2 Ethanol + 2 H_2O + 2 CO_2 + 2 ATP + 2 NADH + 2 H^+

E. Glucose + 3 ADP + 3 P_i → 3 Ethanol + 3 ATP + 3 H_2O

a. A
b. B
c. C
d. D
e. E

Krebs cycle

561. Fill in the gaps of this series:

isocitrate → α-ketoglutarate → _____ → succinate → _____ →malate → acetylCoA + oxaloacetate→ _____

   a. pyruvate / fumarate / lactate
   b. alanine / NADH + H⁺ / citrate
   c. succinylCoA / fumarate / citrate
   d. citrate / succinylCoA / fumarate
   e. FADH₂ / CO₂ / succinylCoA

562. The balanced chemical reaction for a full turn of Krebs cycle is as follows:

   a. AcetylCoA + H_2O + NAD⁺ + 2 FAD + GDP + P_i → 2 CO_2 + NADH + 2 FADH₂ + CoA-SH + GTP
   b. AcetylCoA + 2 H_2O + 3 NAD⁺ + FAD + GDP + P_i → 2 CO_2 + 3 NADH + FADH₂ + CoA-SH + GTP
   c. AcetylCoA + 2 H_2O → 2CO_2
   d. AcetylCoA + 3 NAD⁺ + GDP + P_i → 2 CO_2 + 3 NADH + CoA-SH + GTP
   e. AcetylCoA + 2 H_2O + 4 NAD⁺ + GDP + P_i → 2 CO_2 + 4 NADH + CoA-SH + GTP

563. Citrate synthase catalyzes the adition of acetylCoA to oxaloacetate, producing citrate. How many molecules of CO_2 does a citrate molecule lose across a complete turn of Krebs cycle, until it regenerates citrate again?

   a. 0
   b. 1
   c. 2
   d. 3
   e. 4

564. COMPLETE: in Krebs cycle there are 4 oxidation reactions, in three of them the final acceptor of electrons is _____ and in the other it is _____.

   a. NAD⁺ / FAD
   b. FAD / NAD⁺
   c. FMN / FAD
   d. FAD / FMN
   e. NAD⁺ / FMN

565. Citrate synthase catalyzes the adition of acetylCoA to oxaloacetate, producing citrate. How many molecules of H_2O does a citrate molecule lose across a complete turn of Krebs cycle, until it regenerates citrate again?

    a. 0
    b. 1
    c. 2
    d. 3
    e. 4

566. You have pyruvate labelled by ^{14}C in its carboxylic group, as it's indicated with a star in the following figure,

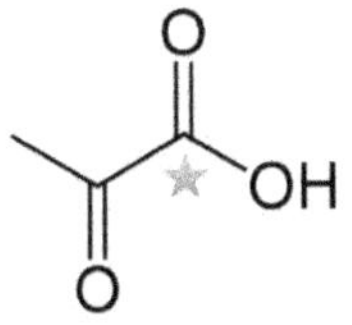

in which molecules could you find the radioactive label after submitting this labelled pyruvate to the action of pyruvate dehydrogenase and one turn of Krebs cycle?

    a. acetylCoA → citrate → isocitrate → α-ketoglutarate → CO_2
    b. acetylCoA → citrate → isocitrate → α-ketoglutarate → succinylCoA → succinate → fumarate → malate → oxaloacetate
    c. acetylCoA → citrate → isocitrate → CO_2
    d. CO_2
    e. acetylCoA → citrate → CO_2

567. Which of the following assertions is FALSE?

    a. Krebs cycle initiates with the adition of two carbon atoms from acetylCoA to oxaloacetate, forming a molecule of 6 carbons named citrate
    b. In several steps, this 6-carbons intermediate loses two molecules of CO_2. The lost carbon atoms are the same that were introduced by the initial acetylCoA
    c. From succinylCoA on, all the main compounds of Krebs cycle, since arriving to oxaloacetate, have 4 carbons
    d. Oxaloacetate, in Krebs cycle, is formed by oxidation of malate, associated to the reduction of a NAD^+ molecule
    e. In Krebs cycle, the adition of an H_2O molecule to fumarate produces malate. This reaction is catalysed by fumarate hydratase

568. If you could label with ^{14}C all the carbon atoms of acetylCoA and follow its path along its first turn across Krebs cycle, what percentage of these atoms will be released as CO_2?

a. 0 %
b. 25 %
c. 50 %
d. 75 %
e. 100 %

569. Fritz Lipmann received, together with Hans Krebs, the Nobel prize in the first half of the 20th century. Krebs was awarded for discovering that some organic compounds degradate in a cyclic route. What was the most known discovery made by Fritz Lipmann?

a. coenzyme A
b. tricarboxylic acids cycle
c. citric acid cycle
d. b and c
e. the anaerobic degradation of pyruvate into lactate

570. Succinate dehydrogenase oxidizes succinate, by forming a double bond between central carbons and generating mainly one of the possible isomers. Which is this molecule?

a. the *cis* isomer of fumarate (also known as maleate)
b. the *trans* isomer of fumarate
c. L-malate
d. D-malate
e. L-oxaloacetate

571. In Krebs cycle, the route from succinate to oxaloacetate goes by the following intermediates...

a. succinate → succinylCoA → fumarate → oxaloacetate
b. succinate → citrate → malate → fumarate → oxaloacetate
c. succinate → malate → fumarate → oxaloacetate
d. succinate → fumarate → malate → oxaloacetate
e. succinate → α-ketoglutarate → malate → oxaloacetate

572. We consider that a GTP and an ATP are interchangeable without any additional energetic cost. So, in the following notations, we'll write only ATP to refer to both. Having this in mind, the complete oxidation of a glucose molecule by glycolysis and Krebs cycle can be summarized with the following chemical equation:

a. Glucose + 10 NAD$^+$ + 4 ADP + 4 P$_i$ → 6 CO_2 + 10 NADH + 4 ATP
b. Glucose + 2 H_2O + 10 NAD$^+$ + 2 FAD + 4 ADP + 4 P$_i$ → 6 CO_2 + 10 NADH + 6 H$^+$ + 2 FADH$_2$ + 4 ATP
c. Glucose + 6 H_2O + 10 NAD$^+$ + 2 FAD + 4 ADP + 4 P$_i$ → 6 CO_2 + 10 NADH + 6 H$^+$ + 2 FADH$_2$ + 4 ATP
d. Glucose + 2 H_2O + 6 NAD$^+$ + 2 FAD + 4 ADP + 4 P$_i$ → 6 CO_2 + 6 NADH + 6 H$^+$ + 2 FADH$_2$ + 2 ATP
e. Glucose + 2 H_2O + 4 NAD$^+$ + 2 FAD + 4 ADP + 4 P$_i$ → 6 CO_2 + 4 NADH + 6 H$^+$ + 2 FADH$_2$ + 4 ATP

573. The cells with an excess of amino acids can transform them into some specific amino acids that, through a 1-step transamination, are directly transformed into Krebs cycle intermediates, in particular α-ketoglutarate and oxaloacetate. Which are these amino acids?

a. alanine and phenylalanine
b. glutamate and aspartate
c. tyrosine and cysteine
d. asparagine and cysteine
e. tyrosine and glycine

574. You have pyruvate labelled by ^{14}C in its central carbon, as it's indicated with a star in the following figure,

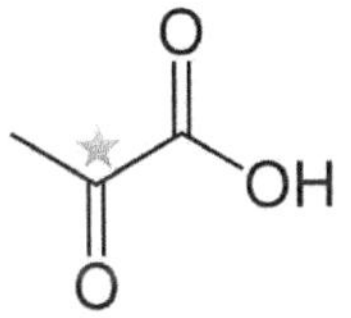

in which molecules could you find the radioactive label after submitting this labelled pyruvate to the action of pyruvate dehydrogenase and one turn of Krebs cycle?

a. acetylCoA → citrate → isocitrate → α-ketoglutarate → CO_2
b. acetylCoA → citrate → isocitrate → α-ketoglutarate → succinylCoA → succinate → fumarate → malate → oxaloacetate
c. acetylCoA → citrate → isocitrate → CO_2
d. CO_2
e. acetylCoA → citrate → CO_2

575. If aconitase (the enzyme that converts citrate into isocitrate) would not asimetrically bind its substrate, what percentage of carbon atoms incorporated to Krebs cycle as acetylCoA would be released in form of CO_2 in a cycle turn?

a. 0 %
b. 25 %
c. 50 %
d. 75 %
e. 100 %

576. In the experiments of Hans Krebs with muscular tissue of pigeon, what effects were observed after adding citrate to this tissue?

a. an increase in pyruvate oxidation proportional to the amount of added citrate
b. a reduction in O_2 consumption proportional to the amount of added citrate
c. a decrease in pyruvate oxidation proportional to the amount of added citrate
d. an increase in O_2 consumption proportional to the amount of added citrate
e. an increase in O_2 consumption extremely high if compared to the amount of added citrate

577. In the experiments of Hans Krebs with muscular tissue of pigeon, which of the following compounds did inhibit pyruvate consumption?

a. isocitrate
b. succinate
c. citrate
d. cis-aconitate
e. malonate

578. COMPLETE: Krebs cycle initiates when a molecule of 2 carbons (____) is combined with one of 4 carbons (____), producing a molecule of 6 carbons (____)

a. fumarate / oxaloacetate / malate
b. fumarate / malate / oxaloacetate
c. acetylCoA / citrate / oxaloacetate
d. acetylCoA / oxaloacetate / citrate
e. pyruvate / malate / citrate

579. Succinate is converted to fumarate in a reaction catalysed by succinate dehydrogenase. Explain the chemical transformation that occurs in this reaction.

    a. a carbonyl group is added to one of the ends of succinate, forming an aldehyde
    b. a carbonyl group is added to one of the central carbons of succinate, forming a ketone
    c. one of the ends of succinate is oxidized, producing a dicarboxylic acid
    d. a dehydrogenation (double bond formation) is produced between the central carbons of succinate
    e. a CO_2 molecule is lost, producing a molecule of 3 carbons

580. Which of the following assertions on the experiments of Hans Krebs with muscle tissue of pigeon is FALSE?

    a. the adition of malonate produced the accumulation of α-ketoglutarate
    b. when adding pyruvate and oxaloacetate, citrate was accumulated
    c. the adition of cis-aconitate produced a decrease in O_2 consumption
    d. when adding malonate, O_2 consumption was stopped
    e. when adding malonate, citrate was accumulated

581. Pyruvate dehydrogenase, in particular its enzymatic activity E_2 (dihydrolipoamide acetyltransferase) is inhibited by one of the following compounds:

    a. acetylCoA
    b. CoA-SH
    c. citrate
    d. pyruvate
    e. succinylCoA

582. Which of these substances do act as coenzymes and are bound to the enzymes of the Pyruvate Dehydrogenase complex?

    a. TPP
    b. FAD
    c. Lipoic acid
    d. a and c
    e. a, b and c

583. In the pass from succinylCoA to succinate, within Krebs cycle, a substrate level phosphorylation occurs. Which is the triphosphate nucleotide most frequently produced into hepatic cells, for example?

a. ATP
b. CTP
c. GTP
d. TTP
e. UTP

584. You have pyruvate labelled with ^{14}C in the non-carboxylic end, as is indicated with a star in the following figure,

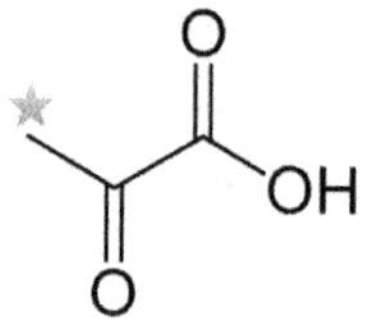

in which molecules could you find the radioactive label after submitting this labelled pyruvate to the action of pyruvate dehydrogenase and one turn of Krebs cycle?

a. acetylCoA → citrate → isocitrate → α-ketoglutarate → CO_2
b. acetylCoA → citrate → isocitrate → α-ketoglutarate → succinylCoA → succinate → fumarate → malate → oxaloacetate
c. acetylCoA → citrate → isocitrate → CO_2
d. CO_2
e. acetylCoA → citrate → CO_2

585. The reaction catalysed by malate dehydrogenase is as follows...

a. L-malate + NAD^+ → oxaloacetate + NADH + H^+
b. D-malate + NAD^+ → oxaloacetate + NADH + H^+
c. L-malate + FAD → oxaloacetate + $FADH_2$
d. D-malate + FAD → oxaloacetate + $FADH_2$
e. L-malate + NAD^+ → citrate + NADH + H^+

586. The conversion of pyruvate into acetylCoA is catalysed by...

    a. phosphofructokinase
    b. la acetylcholinesterase
    c. pyruvate dehydrogenase
    d. lactate dehydrogenase
    e. acyl-CoA transcarbamylase

587. When pyruvate undergoes the chain of reactions catalysed by pyruvate dehydrogenase, which is the destination of its three carbon atoms after this reaction?

    a. 2 pass to CO_2 and 1 to acetylCoA
    b. 2 pass to acetylCoA and 1 is added to oxaloacetate
    c. 2 pass to acetylCoA and 1 incorporates to Krebs cycle
    d. 2 pass to acetylCoA and 1 to CO_2
    e. b and c are right

588. Pyruvate dehydrogenase, in particular its enzymatic activity E_2 (dihydrolipoamide acetyltransferase) is activated by one of these compounds:

    a. acetylCoA
    b. CoA-SH
    c. citrate
    d. pyruvate
    e. succinylCoA

589. If aconitase (the enzyme that converts citrate into isocitrate) would not asimetrically bind its substrate, what percentage of carbon atoms incorporated to Krebs cycle as acetylCoA would be released in form of CO_2 after two cycle turns?

    a. 0 %
    b. 25 %
    c. 50 %
    d. 75 %
    e. 100 %

590. Pyruvate dehydrogenase complex is made of three enzymes...

a. pyruvate dehydrogenase (E_1), dihydrolipoamide dehydrogenase (E_2) and dihydrolipoamide acetyltransferase (E_3)
b. dihydrolipoamide acetyltransferase (E_1), NADH-reductase (E_2) and dihydrolipoamide dehydrogenase (E_3)
c. NADH-reductase (E_1), dihydrolipoamide dehydrogenase (E_2) and dihydrolipoamide acetyltransferase (E_3)
d. pyruvate carboxylase (E_1), dihydrolipoamide acetyltransferase (E_2) and citrate synthase(E_3)
e. pyruvate dehydrogenase (E_1), dihydrolipoamide dehydrogenase (E_2) and citrate synthase (E_3)

591. Pyruvate dehydrogenase (PDH) complex is formed by three enzymes, pyruvate dehydrogenase (E_1), dihydrolipoamide dehydrogenase (E_2) and dihydrolipoamide acetyltransferase (E_3). How many polypeptidic chains of each enzyme does each PDH complex contain in prokaryotes?

a. 1 E_1, 2 E_2 and 1 E_3
b. 24 E_1, 24 E_2 and 12 E_3
c. 12 E_1, 12 E_2 and 6 E_3
d. 6 E_1, 12 E_2 and 12 E_3
e. 6 E_1, 12 E_2 and 6 E_3

592. In the pass from succinylCoA to succinate, within Krebs cycle, a substrate level phosphorylation occurs. Depending on the tissue, succinylCoA synthetase prefers to phosphorylate a different substrate. Which is the triphosphate nucleotide most frequently produced into brain cells, for example?

a. ATP
b. CTP
c. GTP
d. TTP
e. UTP

593. In an experiment, we start from pyruvate labelled with ^{14}C in the non-carboxylic end, as it's indicated with a star in the following figure,

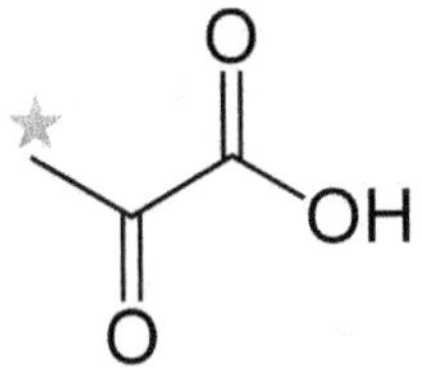

This substrate is added to a cell culture of hepatocytes to which previously have been added high concentrations of malonate (an inhibitor of succinate dehydrogenase). We consider that the concentrations added are enough to block the 100 % of the activity of this enzyme. After some time, samples of metabolites of Krebs cycle are recollected and analyzed, observing that there are isocitrate molecules with two labelled carbons, in particular those shown in this figure.

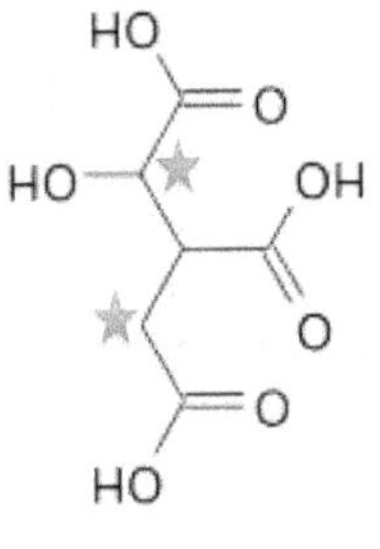

How would you explain this result?

a. since Krebs cycle is not blocked by the blocking of succinate dehydrogenase
b. because, although Krebs cycle is blocked when succinate dehydrogenase is not working, the flux can continue through the Cori's cycle
c. because, although Krebs cycle is blocked when succinate dehydrogenase is not working, the flux can continue through the anaplerotic route catalysed by pyruvate carboxylase
d. because, although Krebs cycle is blocked when succinate dehydrogenase is not working, the flux can continue through the glyoxylate cycle
e. because, although Krebs cycle is blocked when succinate dehydrogenase is not working, the flux can continue through pentose phosphate pathway

594. Which of the following assertions on the regulation of pyruvate dehydrogenase (PDH) complex is FALSE?

a. a high concentration of free Mg^{2+} activates a phosphatase that eliminates the phosphate groups of specific serines within the PDH complex, then activating it
b. a high concentration of free Mg^{2+} is produced when [ATP]/[ADP] relation is low
c. the action of a kinase adds phosphate groups to specific serines of the PDH complex, then inactivating it
d. an increase in [acetylCoA] activates the kinases that add phosphate groups to PDH complex, then inactivating it.
e. an increase in [NADH] activates the kinases that add phosphate groups to PDH complex, then activating it.

595. Pyruvate dehydrogenase (PDH) complex is formed by three enzymes, pyruvate dehydrogenase (E_1), dihydrolipoamide dehydrogenase (E_2) and dihydrolipoamide acetyltransferase (E_3). Which coenzymes do accompany each one of these enzymatic activities?

a. Thiamine pyrophosphate (TPP) is bound to E_1, lipoic acid is bound to E_2 and flavin-adenine dinucleotide (FAD) participates in the reaction of E_3.
b. Nicotine and adenine dinucleotide (NAD) participates in the reaction of E_1, thiamine pyrophosphate (TPP) is bound to E_2 and flavin-adenine dinucleotide (FAD) participates in the reaction of E_3.
c. Coenzyme A (CoA) is bound to E_1, thiamine pyrophosphate is bound to E_2 and lipoic acid participates in the reaction of E_3.
d. Thiamine pyrophosphate (TPP) is bound to E_1, nicotine-adenine dinucleotide (NAD) is bound to E_2 and flavin-adenine dinucleotide (FAD) participates in the reaction of E_3.
e. Lipoic acid is bound to E_1, nicotine-adenine dinucleotide participates in the reaction of E_2 and coenzyme A (CoA) participates in the reaction of E_3.

596. If glucose is completely metabolized through glycolysis and Krebs cycle, which atoms of glucose will be first incorporated into CO_2?

a. 1 and el 2
b. 3 and el 4
c. 5 and el 6
d. 1 and el 4
e. 3 and el 6

597. In which two steps of Krebs cycle is CO_2 produced as residue?

a. acetylCoA + oxaloacetate → citrate ; citrate → isocitrate
b. citrate → isocitrate ; succinylCoA → succinate
c. isocitrate → α-ketoglutarate ; fumarate → malate
d. isocitrate → α-ketoglutarate ; α-ketoglutarate → succinylCoA
e. malate → oxaloacetate ; isocitrate → α-ketoglutarate

598. There is an enzymatic complex within Krebs cycle in which participate the same 5 coenzymes found in the Pyruvate Dehydrogenase Complex. Which is this complex?

a. α-ketoglutarate dehydrogenase
b. isocitrate dehydrogenase
c. aconitasa
d. sucinylCoA sintetasa
e. none of the previous

599. Which of the following assertions is FALSE?

a. Pyruvate dehydrogenase complex of Escherichia coli has a mass higher than 1000 kDa
b. Pyruvate dehydrogenase complex of Escherichia coli is higher than a bacterial ribosome
c. In eukaryotes, the size of the pyruvate dehydrogenase complex approximately doubles that of procaryotes
d. In procaryotes, pyruvate dehydrogenase complex has 60 subunits organized following a cubic symmetry.
e. In eukaryotes, pyruvate dehydrogenase complex has 96 subunits organized following a cubic symmetry.

600. Which of the following conditions will not result in an increase of the velocity of pyruvate dehydrogenase complex?

a. a decrease in [ATP]/[AMP] ratio
b. an increase in [NAD$^+$]/[NADH] ratio
c. an increase in the concentration of CoA-SH (coenzyme A in its reduced form)
d. an increase in the concentration of glucose
e. a decrease in [CoA-SH]/[acetylCoA] ratio

601. Thiamine pyrophosphate (TPP) acts as coenzyme in many decarboxylations of α-ketoacids. Recent NMR studies have elucidated that the role of TPP is to act as a nucleophile that attacks the carbonyl group of these ketoacids, thus allowing the release of a CO_2 molecule. Observe the chemical structure of TPP and answer. Which is the atom of TPP that directly participates in this nucleophilic attack?

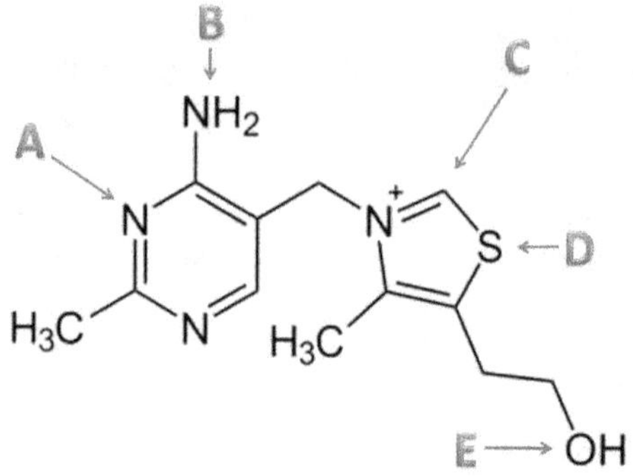

a. A
b. B
c. C
d. D
e. E

602. How does fluoroacetate, a potent pesticide tha inhibits Krebs cycle, acts?

a. It's an inhibitor of citrate synthase, given its similarity to acetylCoA.
b. It's transformed into fluoroacetylCoA, that acts as substrate of citrate synthase, producing fluorocitrate, that inhibits aconitase.
c. It's an iron chelating agent, that avoids the formation of iron-sulphur centers (4Fe – 4S), that are essential for the catalytic action of aconitase
d. It's transformed into fluoroacetylCoA, that is an inhibitor of citrate synthase, since it mimics its substrate, acetylCoA.
e. It deprotonates citrate, strongly reducing its affinity for the active site of aconitase.

603. For thiamine pyrophosphate (TPP) to exert its catalytic role in α-cetoacids decarboxylation, the enzyme that hosts it must remove a proton from it. By which of the following amino acids is most likely for the enzyme to make this task?

a. Glutamic acid
b. Tyrosine
c. Histidine
d. Lysine
e. Alanine

604. Pyruvate dehydrogenase, in particular its enzymatic activity E_3 (dihydrolipoamide dehydrogenase) is inhibited by one of the following compounds:

a. NADH
b. NAD$^+$
c. citrate
d. FADH$_2$
e. acetylCoA

605. Lipoic acid acts as coenzyme in the reaction of the pyruvate dehydrogenase complex. For this, it must be covalently bound to the enzyme. This binding is made by an amide bond between its own carboxylic group and...

a. ...an hydroxyl of serine or threonine (exceptionally, also of tyrosine)
b. ...another carboxylic group of glutamic or aspartic acid
c. ...a δ-amino group of an arginine
d. ...an ε-amino group of a lysine
e. ...a β-amino group of glutamine or asparagine

606. Pyruvate dehydrogenase (PDH) complex catalyzes the following reaction.

a. Pyruvate + CoA + NAD$^+$ $\rightarrow$ acetyl-CoA + CO$_2$ + NADH
b. Pyruvate + NAD$^+$ $\rightarrow$ Lactate + NADH
c. Pyruvate + NADH $\rightarrow$ Lactate + CO$_2$ + NAD$^+$
d. Pyruvate + CoA + NADH $\rightarrow$ acetyl-CoA + CO$_2$ + NAD$^+$
e. Pyruvate + CoA + NAD$^+$ $\rightarrow$ acetyl-CoA + NADH

607. Pyruvate dehydrogenase complex has, among the following compounds, an allosteric inhibitor. Which is it?

    a. AMP
    b. NAD+
    c. phosphoenolpyruvate
    d. pyruvate
    e. α-ketoglutarate

608. Pyruvate dehydrogenase (PDH) complex is formed by three enzymes. Covalently bound to dihydrolipoamide acetyltransferase (E_2) there are two lipoamide residues. Which of the following assertions in relation to the role of these residues is FALSE?

    a. Each lipoamide is bound to the lateral chain of a lysine residue, giving rise to a linear chain of ~1,4 nm of length.
    b. One of the lipoamides directly interacts with hydroxyetil-TPP of the enzyme E_1, covalently binding the ethyl group coming from pyruvate and forming a thioester with it.
    c. Both lipoamides interchange the acetyl residue that they have bound by a thioester.
    d. The adition of reduced CoA results in the reduction of one of the lipoamide groups and the generation of acetylCoA.
    e. Lipoamide group, reduced after the formation of acetylCoA, is oxidized again thus directly delivering its electrons to NAD+ and producing NADH

609. Which is the reaction catalysed by the enzyme citrate synthase?

    a. pyruvate + malate + H_2O → citrate
    b. acetylCoA + H_2O → citrate + CoA
    c. acetylCoA + oxaloacetate + H_2O → citrate + CoA + H+
    d. acetylCoA + fumarate + H_2O → citrate + CoA + H+
    e. pyruvate + oxaloacetate + H_2O → citrate

610. Isocitrate dehydrogenase catalyzes the transformation of isocitrate into α-ketoglutarate. The mechanism of action for this reaction is as follows:

a. Isocitrate is oxidized and, later, a molecule of CO_2 is lost.
b. Isocitrate loses a molecule of CO_2 and, later, it's oxidized to α-ketoglutarate, reducing a molecule of FAD.
c. Isocitrate loses a molecule of CO_2 and, later, it's oxidized to α-ketoglutarate, reducing a molecule of NAD^+
d. Isocitrate is fragmented into two molecules: ethanol (2C) and succinate (4C). A molecule of CO_2 is added to the later, to form α-ketoglutarate.
e. Isocitrate is dehydrated, forming aconitate. This takes again a H_2O molecule, as well as loses a CO_2.

611. In the pass from succinylCoA to succinate, within Krebs cycle, a substrate level phosphorylation occurs. Depending on the tissue, succinylCoA synthetase prefers to phosphorylate a different substrate. Which is the triphosphate nucleotide most frequently produced into cardiac muscle cells, for example?

a. ATP
b. CTP
c. GTP
d. TTP
e. UTP

612. In the reaction of succinylCoA synthetase, an inorganic phosphate (P_i) is covalently added to a residue of the enzyme, releasing reduced coenzymeA. This phosphate is then transferred to GDP to form GTP. Which is this residue?

a. serine
b. tyrosine
c. asparagine
d. glutamine
e. histidine

613. Succinate dehydrogenase catalyzes the oxidation of succinate to fumarate. For this, a molecule of FAD covalently bound to the enzyme is reduced to give rise to $FADH_2$. In order to be again operational, this $FADH_2$ must be again reoxidized. How is this done?

a. It transfers its electrons to pyruvate forming glyceraldehyde
b. It transfers its electrons to the mitochondrial electronic transport chain
c. It transfers its electrons to SO_2 forming SH_2
d. It transfers its electrons to CO_2 para formar CH_4
e. It transfers its electrons to pyruvate forming lactate

614. Glyoxylate cycle...

a. ...needs the catalytic action of the enzymes malate synthase and isocitrate lyase
b. ...allows the microorganisms containing acetate thiokinase (able to convert acetate into acetylCoA) to feed from this acid and make complex sugars
c. ...produces succinate, that must be transported to mitochondria to be converted into oxaloacetate
d. a and b are true
e. a, b and c are true

615. Pyruvate dehydrogenase, in particular its enzymatic activity E_3 (dihydrolipoamide dehydrogenase) is activated by the following compounds:

a. NADH
b. NAD^+
c. citrate
d. $FADH_2$
e. acetylCoA

616. Pyruvate dehydrogenase has, among the following compounds, an allosteric inhibitor. Which is?

a. AMP
b. ATP
c. acetylCoA
d. citrate
e. α-ketoglutarate

617. We call 'anaplerotic routes' to...

a. those metabolic pathways that allow to replace the intermediates of Krebs cycle that have been used in biosynthetic routes
b. those metabolic routes followed by succinate for the biosynthesis of heme group
c. those metabolic routes that, starting from any intermediate of Krebs cycle, go towards the biosynthesis of more complex molecules
d. those metabolic routes that, starting from any intermediate of Krebs cycle, are part of the cellular anabolism
e. c and d are right

618. One of the main anaplerotic routes, specially in liver and kidney of mammals, is catalysed by the enzyme pyruvate carboxylase, which reaction does this enzyme catalyse?

a. the pass from pyruvate to malate
b. the pass from pyruvate to fumarate
c. the pass from pyruvate to acetylCoA
d. the pass from pyruvate to citrate
e. the pass from pyruvate to oxaloacetate

619. Pyruvate carboxylase is alosterically activated by...

a. pyruvate
b. acetylCoA
c. malate
d. oxaloacetate
e. NAD^+

620. Which of the following assertions on glyoxylate cycle is FALSE?

a. It avoids the reactions of Krebs cycle that result in a lost of CO_2
b. It involves the fragmentation of isocitrate (6C) into glyoxylate (2C) and succinate (4C), by the enzyme isocitrate lyase
c. It involves the binding between acetylCoA (2C) and glyoxylate (2C) to form malate, by the enzyme malate synthase
d. Each cycle turn, 2 molecules of acetylCoA are converted into oxaloacetate
e. The succinate produced by isocitrate lyase is driven to glyoxysome, where it's converted into oxaloacetate

621. Pyruvate carboxylase is a tetrameric protein that catalyzes the conversion of pyruvate into oxaloacetate. For this, it uses a coenzyme. CO_2 is added to this coenzyme in a first step. Later, CO_2 is transferred from the coenzyme to pyruvate. This coenzyme acts very often as cofactor in carboxylations in which CO_2 participates. Which is this coenzyme?

a. Coenzyme A
b. NADH
c. TPP
d. Lipoic acid
e. Biotin

622. In bacteria and plants there is an anaplerotic route alternative to pyruvate carboxylase. It is phosphoenolpyruvate carboxylase. Which of the following assertions in relation to this route is TRUE?

a. This enzyme catalyzes conversion of phosphoenolpyruvate into oxaloacetate
b. This enzyme does not use biotin as cofactor
c. It is a route very active within C_4 pathway for CO_2 fixation
d. a and c are right
e. All are right

623. In one of the reactions of glyoxylate cycle, glyoxylate (2C) and succinate (4C) are produced. Glyoxylate is combined with acetylCoA to make malate. Succinate is driven into a cellular organelle, to be transformed into oxaloacetate through 3 reactions of Krebs cycle. Which is this organelle?

a. chloroplast
b. mitochondria
c. glyoxysome
d. peroxisome
e. lysosome

624. The reaction catalysed by the malic enzyme is a known anaplerotic route, which is the balanced equation for this reaction?

a. pyruvate + HCO_3^- + NADPH + H^+ → L-malate + $NADP^+$ + H_2O
b. acetylCoA + 2 HCO_3^- + 2 NADPH + 2 H^+ → L-malate + 2 $NADP^+$ + H_2O
c. acetylCoA + 2 HCO_3^- + 2 NADPH + 2 H^+ → L-malate + 2 $NADP^+$ + 2 H_2O
d. pyruvate + CO_2 + NADH + H^+ → L-malate + NAD^+
e. pyruvate + CO_2 + NADH + H^+ → L-malate + NAD^+ + H_2O

625. Many plants can directly produce sugars from the fats accumulated in their seeds. They do this by using an anabolic variant of Krebs cycle named...

    a. Cori cycle
    b. Hatch-Slach cycle
    c. Calvin cycle
    d. glyoxylate cycle
    e. citric acid cycle

626. Isocitrate lyase catalyzes the following reaction.

    a. isocitrate $\rightarrow$ a-ketoglutarate + CO_2
    b. isocitrate $\rightarrow$ succinate + glyoxylate
    c. isocitrate $\rightarrow$ fumarate + 2 CO_2
    d. isocitrate $\rightarrow$ malate + 2 CO_2
    e. isocitrate + 2 CoA-SH $\rightarrow$ 2 acetylCoA + glyoxylate

627. Malate synthase catalyzes the following reaction.

    a. glyoxylate + acetylCoA + H_2O $\rightarrow$ malate + CoA-SH + H^+
    b. glyoxylate + acetylCoA + NADH + H^+ $\rightarrow$ malate + CoA-SH
    c. glyoxylate + acetylCoA $\rightarrow$ malate + CoA-SH
    d. succinate + H_2O $\rightarrow$ malate
    e. succinate + NAD^+ $\rightarrow$ malate + NADH + H^+

628. The main destination of the succinate produced in glyoxylate cycle is...

    a. the production of acetylCoA, derived to fatty acids synthesis (lipogenesis)
    b. the transformation into several fermentation products, mainly lactate
    c. the oxidation through Krebs cycle and the production of ATP through the electronic transport chain and oxidative phosphorilation
    d. the conversion into oxaloacetate that enters gluconeogenesis
    e. the synthesis of small amino acids

Pentose phosphate pathway

629. Which are the two main metabolic goals of the pentose phosphate pathway?

a. the reduction of the concentration of glucose in the cytosol and the production of components for nucleic acids
b. the generation of NADPH needed for biosynthetic routes and the fabrication of ribose-5-P for the biosynthesis of nucleotides
c. the generation of α-ketoglutarate for amino acid biosynthesis and the production of ribose-5-P for nucleotide biosynthesis
d. the reduction of the concentration of glucose in the cytosol and the generation of NADPH needed for biosynthetic routes
e. the fabrication of NADPH to be used in gluconeogenesis and the fabrication of ribulose-5-P for heme group synthesis

630. Pentose phosphate pathway can be a good route for the metabolization of riboses coming from diet. In which molecules do we mainly find these residues?

a. nucleic acids
b. triglycerides
c. steroids
d. sugars
e. proteins

631. Pentose phosphate pathway has an starting oxidative phase in which glucose-6-phosphate is oxidized into 6-phosphogluconolactone, then oxidized to 6-phosphogluconate that, in turn, is oxidized and decarboxylated until forming ribulose-5-phosphate. For each mole of glucose-6-phosphate the enters this step, finally we obtain...

a. one mole of NADPH, one mole of CO_2 and one mole of ribulose-5-phosphate
b. two moles of NADPH, two moles of CO_2 and one mole of ribulose-5-phosphate
c. two moles of NADPH, one mole of CO_2 and one mole of ribulose-5-phosphate
d. two moles of NADPH, one mole of CO_2 and two moles of ribulose-5-phosphate
e. one mole of NADPH and one mole of ribulose-5-phosphate

632. In the following simplified scheme of pentose phosphate pathway, A, B, C and D letters must be substituted by...

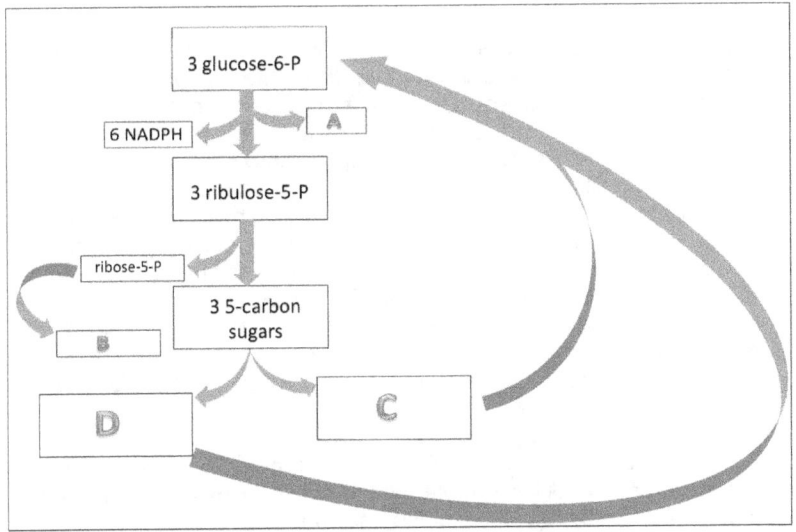

a. A='3 CO_2' / B='heme group' / C='2 ribose-5-P' / D='4 acetylCoA'

b. A='3 CO_2' / B='heme group' / C=' 2 six-carbon sugars' / D=' 1 three-carbon sugar'

c. A='2 acetylCoA' / B='nucleotides' / C='1 three-carbon sugar' / D='2 6-carbon sugars'

d. A='3 CO_2' / B='nucleotides' / C='1 three-carbon sugar' / D='2 six-carbon sugars'

e. A='2 CO_2' / B='nucleotides' / C='1 three-carbon sugar' / D='1 six-carbon sugar'

633. Pentose phosphate pathway has a first oxidative phase where ribulose-5-phosphate is produced. This metabolite is then isomerized to ribose-5-phosphate, which is used in the synthesis of nucleic acids components. When this synthesis is not needed, ribose-5-phosphate must be metabolized. How is this perfomed?

a. By a complex series of reactions, three riboses-5-P are converted into two six-carbon sugars and a three-carbon sugar, that enter the glycolytic pathway.
b. By a complex series of reactions, two riboses-5-P are converted into a six-carbon sugar and a four-carbon sugar. The hexose enters the glycolytic pathway and the tetrose is finally incorporated into Krebs cycle.
c. By a complex series of reactions, four riboses-5-P are converted into three six-carbon sugars and a molecule of acetylCoA. The hexoses enter the glycolytic pathway and the acetylCoA is finally incorporated into Krebs cycle.
d. By a complex series of reactions, three riboses-5-P are converted into a six-carbon sugar and two three-carbon sugars, which enter glycolytic pathway.
e. By a complex series of reactions, three riboses-5-P are converted into a six-carbon sugar, which enters the glycolytic pathway, and two succinate molecules that are incorporated into Krebs cycle. In the process, two molecules of CO_2 are lost.

634. Glucose-6-P dehydrogenase deficiency is a genetic X-linked disease that affects to more than 400 million people. Which of the following situations is a clear consequence of extremely low levels of this enzyme?

a. The endogenous synthesis of nucleic acids is blocked, and the person dies by his/her incapacity of regenerating the cardiac muscular tissue.
b. Gluthatione within erythrocytes loses its ability for being reduced, since this process needs almost exclusively of the NADPH produced in the pentose phosphate pathway. This makes that erythrocytes cannot maintain their hemoglobin in a reduced state (Fe^{2+}), besides causing hemolysis in conditions of oxidative stress, as those derived from infections or the ingestion of certain drugs.
c. Glucose-6-P cannot be introduced into pentose phosphate pathway and it accumulates, producing crystals of a reduced form of glucose (sorbitol) specially visible in the crystalline lens of the eye.
d. Fatty acids production from sugars is almost blocked, thus generating a huge increase in glycogen storage that appears as an hepatomegaly.
e. Derivation of glucose towards heme group synthesis is almost blocked, so erythrocytes cannot be renewed, thus producing common anemia symptoms.

Electron transport chain and oxidative phosphorylation

635. If a glucose molecule is completely oxidized, yielding 38 ATPs, and needing for this oxidation to participate in the mitochondrial electron transport chain, the final acceptor of its electrons is...

a. NADH + H$^+$
b. FADH$_2$
c. coenzyme Q
d. O$_2$
e. a and b are right

636. Oxidative phosphorylation entails...

a. the oxidation of H$_2$O to form O$_2$
b. the oxidation of O$_2$ to form H$_2$O
c. the oxidation of H$_2$O to form O$_2$
d. the oxidation of O$_2$ to form H$_2$O
e. none of the previous

637. Chemiosmotic hypothesis was formulated by...

a. Peter Mitchell
b. Claude Bernard
c. Max Perutz
d. Carl Ferdinand Cori
e. Stanley Miller

638. As chemiosmotic hypothesis outlines...

a. the differences in proton concentrations at both sides of the inner mitochondrial membrane are the manifestation of the energy obtained from the oxidation of sugars, lipids and proteins.
b. the stability of DNA molecule is determined by the concentration of Na$^+$ ions in the major and minor grooves.
c. the differences between the concentrations of Na$^+$ and K$^+$ at both sides of plasma membrane determine the generation of an action potential and, so, the transmission of nervous signal.
d. the rate of glycolytic pathway is affected by H$^+$ concentration, that is, by pH
e. the affinity of hemoglobin by O$_2$ is affected by H$^+$ concentration, that is, by pH

639. NAD-related dehydrogenases withdrawtwo hydrogen atoms from their substrates. One of them is transferred as _____ to NAD^+, and another is transferred as _____ to the environment.

a. hydride anion / hydride anion
b. proton / proton
c. hydride cation / hydride cation
d. hydride cation / proton
e. hydride anion / proton

640. The transfer of electrons from $FADH_2$ or from NADH has a basic difference...

a. NADH is a larger molecule and, so, its redox potential is higher than that of $FADH_2$
b. $FADH_2$ is a soluble electron transporter and its chemical environment (aqueous solution) does not vary es un transportador de electrones soluble and su entorno químico (disolución acuosa) no varía so much as that of NADH, so its redox potential is more constant and that of NADH is more variable
c. $FADH_2$ is normally strongly bound to flavoproteins, so its redox potential considerably varies as a result of the closest protein residues. As NADH generally is in soluble form, it does not have this variable behaviour.
d. $FADH_2$ is a larger molecule and, so, its redox potential is higher than that of NADH.
e. NADH only transfers protons, whereas $FADH_2$ can transfer hydride anions

641. Cytochromes...

a. a and b have the heme group covalently bound
b. a and c have the heme group covalently bound
c. a and b have the heme group tightly bound, but not in a covalent form
d. b and c have the heme group tightly bound, but not in a covalent form
e. a and c have the heme group tightly bound, but not in a covalent form

642. Who discovered that mitochondria were the place where oxidative phosphorylation takes occurs?

a. Peter Mitchell and Stanley Pawson
b. Albert Lehninger and Eugene Kennedy
c. Max Peruzt and Andy Rossman
d. Carl Ferdinand Cori and Gerty Cori
e. Stanley Miller and John Urey

643. Which of the following structures does correspond to ubiquinone?

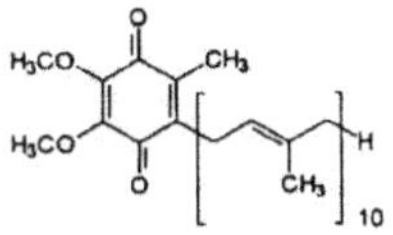

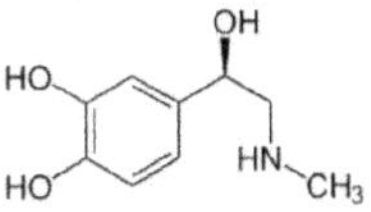

a. A
b. B
c. C
d. D
e. E

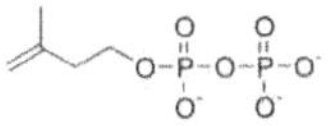

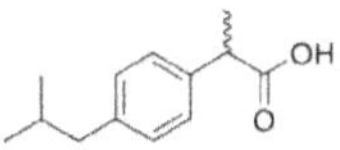

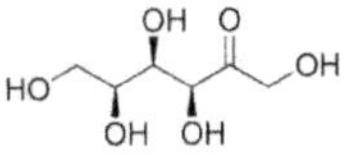

644. External mitochondrial membrane would be permeable to...

a. a molecule of 3 daltons
b. a molecule of 1000 daltons
c. a molecule of 4 kDaltons
d. a and b are right
e. a, b and c are right

645. Which of the following processes does not occur within mitochondrial matrix?

a. β-oxidation of fatty acids
b. pyruvate dehydrogenase reaction
c. glycolysis
d. Krebs cycle
e. routes for the terminal oxidation of amino acids

646. How many complexes of electron transport chain + ATP synthase tend to be in an standard mitochondria of an standard hepatocyte?

a. 1
b. ~10-20
c. ~50-80
d. ~10000
e. millions

647. Mitochondria of the following cells, generally differ when it comes to the number of complexes of electron transport chain + ATP synthase that they hold in theirinner mitochondrial membrane. In the following list, which are the mitochondria where these complexes are most abundant?

a. the mitochondria of hepatocytes
b. the mitochondria of cardiac muscular cells
c. the mitochondria of erythrocytes
d. the mitochondria of intestine bacteria (_Escherichia coli_)
e. the mitochondria of mouth bacteria (_Streptococcus mutans_)

648. To which molecules do the following chemical structures correspond?

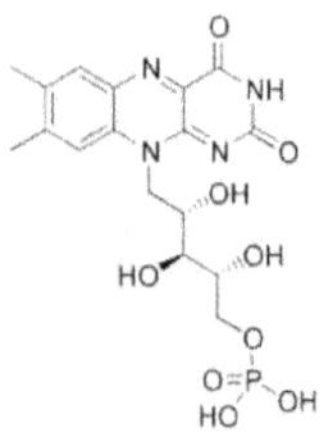

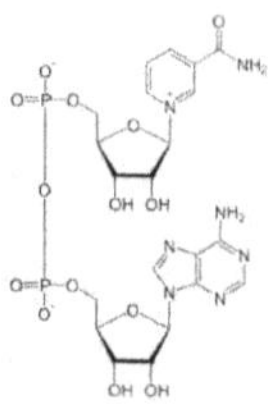

a. A = FAD ; B = FMN ; C = NAD
b. A = NAD ; B = FMN ; C = NAD
c. A = FMN ; B = NAD ; C = FAD
d. A = FAD ; B = NAD ; C = FMN
e. A = FMN ; B = FAD ; C = NAD

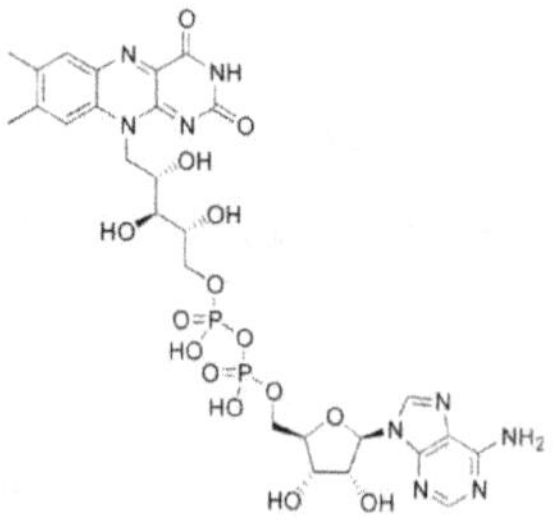

649. The notation 'cytochrome b₅₆₂' indicates...

a. that this cytochrome has 5 molecules of heme group A bound, 6 of heme group B and 2 of heme group C
b. that this cytochrome was discovered as the number 562 among the more than thousand known cytochromes
c. that this cytochrome has a molecular weight of 562 kDa
d. that this cytochrome has a molecular weight of 562 Da
e. that this cytochrome has a maximum of absortion at a wavelength of 562 nm

650. Rieske Fe-S proteins...

a. ...are proteins with Fe-S centers where two of the Fe^{2+} atoms are coordinated to a selenocysteine instead of being bound to a cysteine
b. ...are proteins with Fe-S centers where two of the Fe^{2+} atoms are coordinated to a methionine instead of being bound to a cysteine
c. ...are proteins with Fe-S centers where two of the Fe^{2+} atoms are coordinated to a lysine instead of being bound to a cysteine
d. ...are proteins with Fe-S centers where two of the Fe^{2+} atoms are coordinated to a histidine instead of being bound to a cysteine
e. ...are proteins with Fe-S centers where two of the Fe^{2+} atoms are coordinated to a tyrosine instead of being bound to a cysteine

651. The following picture...

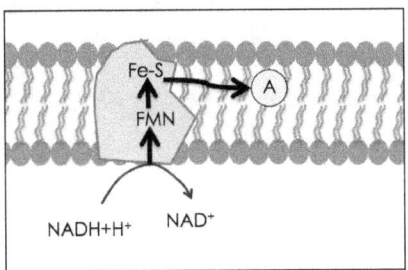

a. ...represents the complex II of the mitochondrial electron transport chain, the letter A refers to ubiquinone
b. ......represents the complex I of the mitochondrial electron transport chain, the letter A refers to ubiquinone
c. ......represents the complex I of the mitochondrial electron transport chain, the letter A refers to a Rieske center
d. ......represents the complex II of the mitochondrial electron transport chain, the letter A refers to coenzyme Q
e. ......represents the complex I of the mitochondrial electron transport chain, the letter A refers to ubiquinone 2Fe-2S center

652. NADH dehydrogenase...

a. is the first enzyme (complex I) of mitochondrial electron transport chain
b. is the second enzyme (complex II) of mitochondrial electron transport chain
c. is the third enzyme (complex III) of mitochondrial electron transport chain
d. is the fourth enzyme (complex IV) of mitochondrial electron transport chain
e. is the fifth enzyme (complex V) of mitochondrial electron transport chain

Other reactions of oxygen in the body

653. We use the term oxidase to refer to enzymes that...

a. ...catalyse the oxidation of a substrate by the addition of one of the oxygen atoms of O_2 to the product.
b. ...catalyse the oxidation of a substrate without adding any of the oxygen atoms of O_2 to the product
c. ...catalyse the oxidation of a substrate by the reduction of the coenzyme FAD
d. ...catalyse the oxidation of a substrate by the reduction of NADH coenzyme
e. ...catalyse the oxidation of a substrate by generating H_2O_2

654. An enzyme that catalyzes reactions that correspond to a generic equation like...
$$A\text{-}H + BH_2 + O=O \rightarrow A\text{-}OH + B + H_2O$$
...which name does receive?

a. oxidases
b. hydratases
c. monooxygenases
d. peroxidases
e. dioxygenases

655. We use the term oxygenase to refer to enzymes that...

a. ...catalyse the oxidation of a substrate by the addition of one of the oxygen atoms of O_2 to the product.
b. ...catalyse the oxidation of a substrate without adding any of the oxygen atoms of O_2 to the product
c. ...catalyse the oxidation of a substrate by the reduction of the coenzyme FAD
d. ...catalyse the oxidation of a substrate by the reduction of NADH coenzyme
e. ...catalyse the oxidation of a substrate by generating H_2O_2

656. All cytochromes P$_{450}$ share a common structural feature, which is it?

a. Six a-helices surround the heme group
b. The two positions of heme group not bound to porphyrin are occupied by aspartate residues, that move away in presence of O_2 or carbon monoxide, to allow the coordination of these gases
c. One of the coordination positions of the heme group has an ionized cupper atom (Cu^{2+}) constitutively bound, what entails that these proteins may intensely absorb light at 450 nm
d. One of the six coordination positions of heme group is occupied by the thiolate ion of a cysteine
e. They present 4 hydroxyproline residues covalently bound to heme group

657. The enzyme superoxide dismutase catalyzes the following reaction:

a. $4\,OH \cdot \rightarrow 2\,H_2O + O_2$
b. $O_2 \cdot^- + OH \cdot + H^+ \rightarrow H_2O + O_2$
c. $O_2 \cdot^- + H_2O_2 \cdot^- + 2\,H^+ \rightarrow 2\,H_2O + O_2$
d. $2\,O_2 \cdot^- \rightarrow 2\,O_2$
e. $2\,O_2 \cdot^- + 2\,H^+ \rightarrow H_2O_2 + O_2$

658. Which of the following assertions on P$_{450}$ cytochromes is FALSE?

a. They add to any one of their substrates two oxygen atoms from O_2 molecule
b. One of the six coordination positions of heme group is occupied by the thiolate ion of a cysteine
c. They are generally found in the endoplasmic reticulum of eukaryotic cells and not in mitochondrias
d. The are involved in the hydroxylation of many compounds, such as the intermediates of steroid hormones biosynthesis
e. The heme group of these proteins, when it's in a reduced form and bound to carbon monoxide, intensely absorbs visible light of a wavelength of 450 nm

659. Where do the oxygen atoms present in hydroxyl groups added to cytochrome P$_{450}$ substrates come from?

a. From O_2
b. From H_2O
c. From H_2O_2
d. From carbon monoxide
e. From soluble iron oxides (FeO, Fe$_2$O)

660. Which is the usual electron donor in cytochrome P_{450} reactions?

a. The thiolate ion of the cysteine coordinated to heme group
b. $NADH + H^+$
c. $FADH_2$
d. $NADPH + H^+$
e. The iron bound to heme group (Fe^{2+})

661. The hydroxylation of substrates by cytochrome P_{450} entails the breaking of an O_2 molecule into two oxygen atoms. One of tehm will be incorporated into the hydroxyl group added to the substrate. Where does the other usually go?

a. It is retained by cytochrome P_{450} and incorporates to other substrate, forming a new hydroxyl group
b. To a molecule of CO_2
c. To a molecule of H_2O_2
d. To a varied series of reactive oxygen species
e. To a molecule of H_2O

662. The electron interchanges between the transporters of one electron and the transporters of two are not 100 % efficient, so frequently species that contain uncompletely reduced oxygen (oxidation state higher than -2) are generated and they are more reactive than O_2. They're known as reactive oxygen species (ROS). Which of the following species are included into this category?

a. hydrogen peroxide (H_2O_2)
b. superoxide ion ($O_2.^-$)
c. hydroxyl radical ($OH \cdot$)
d. b and c are right
e. all are right

663. Hydroxyl radical damages biological membranes by a known chain reaction. Which is it?

a. The formation of volatile aldehydes from membrane phospholipids
b. The formation of peroxide radicals from fatty acids
c. The hydrolysis of membrane phospholipids and their unsolubilization
d. The oxidation of the terminal hydroxyl group from cholesterol molecules
e. The saponification of membrane complex lipids

664. One of the pathological actions of hydroxyl radicals is the production of modified nucleobases (8-oxoguanine, isoguanine,...) If the varying chemical groups aren't directly involved in Watson Crick pairings, why are these changes mutagenic?

   a. Because they weaken the sugar-phosphate backbone of DNA and it breaks.
   b. Since the chemical modifications change the tautomeric preferences and the fidelity of the bases to the amino-oxo tautomers, thus enabling alternative pairings to Watson Crick ones, giving rise to transversions or transitions.
   c. Because base dipoles are altered, and thus the stacking interactions, that drives the selectivity found in Watson Crick pairings, are modified.
   d. Because the flexibility of sugar-base bond is highly modified, allowing the prevalence of those nucleotide conformations that prefer alternative pairings.
   e. Since the bases become more soluble and DNA depolymerisation is more favoured from a thermodynamic point of view.

665. The radical superoxide ($O_2 \cdot \bar{\ }$) isn't toxic by itself but it acquires this toxic ability when combined with another free radical very often produced in animal tissues. It's...

   a. nitric oxide ($NO \cdot$)
   b. hydroxyl radical ($OH \cdot$)
   c. methyl radical ($CH_3 \cdot$)
   d. hydrogen peroxide (H_2O_2)
   e. cyanide radical ($CN \cdot$)

666. The combination of superoxide ion ($O_2 \cdot \bar{\ }$) with nitric oxide ($NO \cdot$) produces a reactive oxygen species called peroxynitrite ($OONO^-$) that causes lipid peroxidation and has an important damaging effect on membrane proteins. Which is this effect?

   a. The oxidation of every disulfide bridge and then protein denaturalization
   b. The reduction of carbonyl groups, causing the break of many peptide bonds
   c. The nitration of hydroxyl groups of tyrosines
   d. The reduction of heterocycles, avoiding the formation of many stacking interactions between aromatic amino acids, then causin protein denaturalization
   e. The protonation of negatively charged amino acids, drastically modifying protein interaction networks

667. There are many non-proteic substances acting as antioxidants in the human body. Which of the following do fulfill this role?
A. gluthatione
B. vitamin C (ascorbic acid)
C. vitamin E (α-tocopherol)
D. uric acid
    a. all
    b. only A, B and C
    c. only A
    d. only A and C
    e. only A and B

668. Among the following antioxidant substances, there is one that acts mainly within the cytoplasm of eukaryotic cells, where it is much more abundant than outside the cell. Which is this substance?
    a. gluthatione
    b. vitamin C (ascorbic acid)
    c. vitamin E (α-tocopherol)
    d. uric acid
    e. β-carotene

669. Among the following antioxidant substances, there is one that acts mainly outside the cell, where it is much more abundant than within the cytoplasm of eukaryotic cells. Which is this substance?
    a. gluthatione
    b. vitamin C (ascorbic acid)
    c. vitamin E (α-tocopherol)
    d. uric acid
    e. β-carotene

670. Among the following antioxidant substances, there is one that acts mainly binding to peroxynitrite and inactivating it. Which is this substance?
    a. gluthatione
    b. vitamin C (ascorbic acid)
    c. vitamin E (α-tocopherol)
    d. uric acid
    e. β-carotene

671. Among the following antioxidant substances, there is one (or more) that acts mainly binding to biological membranes, thus avoiding lipid peroxidation to occur. Which is this substance?
    a. gluthatione
    b. vitamin C (ascorbic acid)
    c. vitamin E (α-tocopherol)
    d. uric acid
    e. b y c

Glycogen metabolism and its regulation

672. Glycogen of an hepatocyte is stored in form of rossettes...

a. in the soluble fraction of cytoplasm
b. in glycosomes
c. in glyoxysomes
d. within smooth endoplasmic reticulum
e. in several endosomes

673. Glycogen phosphorylase releases glucose-1-phosphate. How many oxygen atoms does this monosaccharide have?

a. 5
b. 6
c. 7
d. 8
e. 9

674. Glycogen, for humans, constitute...

a. ~2% of muscular mass and ~10% of liver mass
b. ~10% of muscular mass and ~10% of liver mass
c. ~25% of muscular mass and ~10% of liver mass
d. ~25% of muscular mass and ~50% of liver mass
e. ~10% of muscular mass and ~50% of liver mass

675. Debranching enzyme has a transferase-type enzymatic activity that allows to move a group of ____ glucose residues from near an α-1→6 end to an α-1→4 end. How many residues are?

a. 2
b. 3
c. 4
d. 5
e. 6

676. Glycogen synthase cannot initiate glycogen synthesis from scratch. It needs a small polymer of glucoses that acts as primer, on which more glucoses are added. How many glucoses needs to have this primer at least?

a. 2
b. 4
c. 8
d. 16
e. 32

677. Glycogen synthase cannot initiate glycogen synthesis from scratch. It needs a small polymer of glucoses that acts as primer, on which more glucoses are added. Which protein does catalyse the formation and conservation of this primer?

a. transglycosylase
b. UDP-glucose polymerase
c. glucogenin
d. branching enzyme
e. phosphoglycopolymerase

678. In the liver, glucose-6-phosphate is converted into glucose and sent to blood. This reaction is catalysed by glucose-6-phosphatase. In which cell zone is this enzyme mainly found?

a. in the soluble fraction of cytoplasm
b. in the nucleus
c. in mitochondria
d. within endoplasmic reticulum
e. bound to glycogen rossettes

679. Which of the following assertions is/are FALSE?

a. the more phosphorylated glycogen synthase is, the more active it is
b. the more phosphorylated glycogen phosphorylase is, the more inactive it is
c. the more phosphorylated glycogen synthase is, the more inactive it is
d. the more phosphorylated glycogen phosphorylase is, the more active it is
e. a and b

680. Insulin...

a. increases glucose intake by por los myocytes and adipocytes, by causing the migration of GLUT4 receptor of these cells to the membrane
b. stimulates glycogenesis in liver and muscle
c. inhibits glycogenesis in liver and muscle
d. a and b
e. a and c

681. The substrate of glucogenin is...

a. insulin
b. glucagon
c. adrenaline
d. UDP-glucose
e. AMP_c

Gluconeogenesis

682. One of the following ranges of glucose concentrations in human blood could be considered a normal value of blood sugar (not indicative of problems)?

a. 10-30 mg/dl
b. 80-100 mg/dl
c. 140-160 mg/dl
d. 190-210 mg/dl
e. 240-260 mg/ml

683. During intense exercise, glycogen reservoir of the muscle is mobilized. Glucose is then rapidly and anaerobically oxidized producing an excess of lactate, that is sent to blood. Which is the main destination of this lactate, in quantitative terms?

a. It is captured again by muscle and converted into glucose. It waits to be oxidized by glycolysis, Krebs cycle and respiratory chain, when aerobic oxidation be possible.
b. It goes to liver, and is transformed first into pyruvate, and after into glucose, that is sent to blood and taken by muscle to restore glycogen reservoir.
c. It goes to liver, where it's introduced into Krebs cycle and produces reducing power in form of NADH.
d. It goes to kidney, and is transformed first into pyruvate, and after into alanine or glutamine, by specific transaminases, and it's used in the biosynthesis of amino acids in the kidney.
e. It goes to brain, where it's converted into ketone bodies and is oxidized.

684. The degradation of some amino acids and fatty acids with an odd number of carbons generates some gluconeogenic precursors, which are these molecules?

a. lactate
b. propionyl-CoA
c. acetate
d. acetylCoA
e. ketone bodies

685. Which of the following assertions does most fit with the values of glucose consumption in a healthy person?

a. The brain consumes daily a quantity of glucose generally lower than 10% of the total amount consumed by the whole body.
b. The brain consumes daily ~10 Kg of glucose, that is too much when compared to the ~12 Kg daily consumed by the whole organism, brain included.
c. The brain consumes daily ~15000 mg of glucose, that is too much when related to the ~20000 mg daily consumed by the whole organism, brain included.
d. The brain consumes daily ~120 g of glucose, that is too much when related to the ~160 g daily consumed by the whole organism, brain included.
e. The human brain daily consumes approximately its mass in glucose (~1,3 Kg), while the rest of the body fulfills its requirements with only 500 additional grams

686. The catabolism of fats can generate a net yield of glucose. Which products of this catabolism do allow a net flux of glucose synthesis?

a. propionyl-CoA coming from the β-oxidation of fatty acids with an odd number of carbons
b. glycerol
c. acetylCoA coming from β-oxidation
d. a and b
e. all the previous

687. In an average adult person, how much glucose can be available for a fast usage if we have into account the glucose present in soluble form in body fluids and the glucose coming from the fast degradation of glycogen reservoirs? *De novo* glucose synthesis by gluconeogenesis is excluded.

a. 200 g
b. 2.5 Kg
c. 5 g
d. 20 Kg
e. 800 g

688. The reservoirs of glucose in the body (including soluble glucose and glycogen) amount to a quantity X. Daily consumption of glucose in the body amounts to a quantity Y. If a person in a fasting state would not perfom gluconeogenesis to restore the consumed glucose reserves. How long would it take for this person to deplete these reserves?

a. 1 day
b. 3-4 days
c. 1 week
d. 1 month
e. 1 year

689. The custom of giving whisky to people that are recovering from conditions of cold and humidity can turn counter-productive, why?

a. since ethanol activates gluconeogenesis, and glucose can accumulate forming crystals in the nervous system
b. because ethanol, when it is oxidized in the liver by alcohol dehydrogenase, unbalances the quotient [NADH]/[NAD$^+$], indirectly generating hypoglycemia, that affects to the nervous centers of temperature control, eventually causing a body cooling
c. because ethanol degradation in several tissues, mainly in the liver, generates an excess of NAD$^+$, that stimulates glycolytic pathway, slowing gluconeogenesis. This indirectly generates hypoglycemia, that affects to the nervous centers of temperature control, eventually causing a body cooling
d. since hepatocytes carboxylate a certain proportion of ethanol, converting it into propanol, that finally forms propionyl-CoA in some zones of the medulla oblongata responsible for thermal control. This propionyl-CoA, when incorporated into gluconeogenesis, generates an transitory hypoglycemia that diminishes the amount of signals sent by these nervous centers, generally resulting in a body cooling.
e. because the specific heat of ethanol is lower than that of water, thus complicating the ability of the blood (and other body fluids) to retain heat.

690. Among the following list of compounds, which are frequently used as gluconeogenesis substrates?
A. AcetylCoA in the tissues where glyoxylate cycle is working
B. CO_2 coming from pyruvate dehydrogenase and Krebs cycle
C. Lactate coming from glycolysis
D. Glycerol coming from fats hydrolysis
E. Amino acids coming from diet or protein degradation
F. Propanoate coming from some fatty acid degradations

    a. All
    b. All but B and D
    c. All but B
    d. All but D and F
    e. All but A

691. In which cell compartment(s) does gluconeogenesis take place?

    a. Mitochondria
    b. Endoplasmic reticulum
    c. Mitochondria and glyoxysomes
    d. Mitochondria and peroxisomes
    e. Cytosol

692. The main gluconeogenic organ of human body is _____. In a second place we find _____.

    a. Spleen / Bone marrow
    b. Liver / Renal cortex
    c. Liver / Skeletal striated muscle
    d. Skeletal striated muscle / Liver
    e. Sangre / Kidneys

693. The fatty acids degradated until acetylCoA can continue this route towards glucose synthesis, which requisite is needed for this?

a. That acetylCoA can access as substrate to glyoxylate cycle
b. That acetylCoA may enter Krebs cycle, be converted into CO_2 and, by means of Calvin's cycle, glucose be produced
c. That acetylCoA may be converted into pyruvate by pyruvate dehydrogenase and glycolytic pathway initiate
d. That acetylCoA may be converted into glucose by acetate polymerase
e. That acetylCoA may be converted into succinylCoA by an specific transferase and, through the Cori's cycle, may be transformed into a gluconeogenic substrate of 3 or 4 carbons

694. In many ruminant animals, cellulose degradation produces large amounts of glucose that are to some extent fermented before being absorbed. This generates propanoate and lactate in large amounts. These compounds are incorporated into gluconeogenesis. How does propanoate do this?

a. It is directly dehydrogenated to pyruvate.
b. It is carboxylated giving rise to malate that, through some steps of Krebs cycle, results in oxaloacetate.
c. It is converted into propionyl-CoA. To it a CO_2 is added producing methylmalonylCoA. It isomerizes to form succinylCoA that, through some steps of Krebs cycle, produces oxaloacetate.
d. It is reduced to glycerol, being after transformed to dihydroxyacetone phosphate.
e. It is converted into acetate, then to acetylCoA that, through some steps of Krebs cycle, results in oxaloacetate.

695. Which of the following steps is NOT included in gluconeogenesis pathway?

a. pyruvate → lactate
b. pyruvate → phosphoenolpyruvate
c. glucose-6-P → glucose
d. fructose-1,6-bisP → fructose-6-P
e. oxaloacetate → phosphoenolpyruvate

696. The degradation of amino acids and fatty acids with an odd number of carbons produces propionyl-CoA residues, that go to gluconeogenesis. How is this done?

    a. It's converted into lactate, then to pyruvate and then to phosphoenolpyruvate
    b. It's converted into acetylCoA and then to oxaloacetate
    c. It's converted into succinylCoA and then to oxaloacetate
    d. It's oxidized to propanoate, then to pyruvate & then to phosphoenolpyruvate
    e. It's oxidized to glycerol-3-phosphate and then to dihydroxyacetone phosphate

697. Pyruvate carboxylase is a very important enzyme of gluconeogenesis. Which reaction does it catalyse?

    a. Pyruvate + CO_2 + H_2O + ADP + P_i → oxaloacetate + ATP + 2 H^+
    b. Pyruvate + 3 CO_2 + 3 H_2O + 3 ATP → fructose-1,6-bisP + 3 ADP + 3 P_i + 6 H^+
    c. Pyruvate + H_2O + ADP + P_i → acetate + CO_2+ ATP
    d. Pyruvate + CO_2 + H_2O + ATP → oxaloacetate + ADP + P_i + 2 H^+
    e. Pyruvate + CO_2 → malate

698. Pyruvate carboxylase produces oxaloacetate from pyruvate within mitochondria. For this oxaloacetate to follow the gluconeogenic pathway, it's necessary that it may pass from mitochondria to cytosol. How is this achieved?

    a. By an specific transporter for oxaloacetate, in antiport transport with sodium.
    b. Being previously transformed into succinylCoA, that leaves mitochondria by acylCoA translocase, and being again oxidized to oxaloacetate through three steps within the cytosol, by succinylCoA dehydrogenase, an aromatase and malate dehydrogenase.
    c. By an specific transporter for oxaloacetate, in simport transport with sodium.
    d. Being reduced to malate by mitochondrial malate dehydrogenase. Leaving mitochondria by malate transporter, in an antiport transport with phosphate, and being oxidized to oxaloacetate by a cytosolic malate dehydrogenase.
    e. By an specific transporter for oxaloacetate, in antiport transport with calcium.

699. When the oxaloacetate produced by pyruvate carboxylase arrives to cytosol, the enzyme phosphoenolpyruvate carboxikinase (PEPCK) continues gluconeogenic pathway by transforming it into phosphoenolpyruvate. For this the enzyme needs to phosphorylate it. Which triphosphate nucleotide does it use?

    a. ATP
    b. CTP
    c. GTP
    d. TTP
    e. UTP

700. When the oxaloacetate produced by pyruvate carboxylase arrives to cytosol, phosphoenolpyruvate carboxikinase (PEPCK) continues gluconeogenic pathway by converting it into phosphoenolpyruvate. Which gas is released in this reaction?

    a. O_2
    b. CO_2
    c. N_2
    d. H_2
    e. CO

701. In quantitative terms, which is the most important gluconeogenic precursor in the human body?

    a. glycerol
    b. alanine
    c. lactate
    d. propionyl-CoA
    e. glycine

702. Starting from pyruvate until arrive to glucose, gluconeogenesis has successive steps. Some of them are catalysed by enzymes that can function reversibly in glycolysis. Other, contrarily, do not use glycolytic enzymes and allow to avoid steps of glycolysis that are irreversible. Which of the following gluconeogenesis reactions do belong to this second group?

A   Pyruvate + CO_2 + ATP + H_2O → oxaloacetate + P_i + 2 H^+

B   Oxaloacetate + GTP → phosphoenolpyruvate + CO_2 + GDP

C   Phosphoenolpyruvate + H_2O → 2-phosphoglycerate

D   2-phosphoglycerate → 3-phosphoglycerate

E   3-phosphoglycerate + ATP → 1,3-bisphosphoglycerate + ADP

F   1,3-bisphosphoglycerate + NADH + H^+ → glyceraldehyde-3-P + NAD^+ + P_i

G   Glyceraldehyde-3-P → dihydroxyacetone phosphate

H   Glyceraldehyde-3-P + dihydroxyacetone phosphate → fructose-1,6-bisP

I   Fructose-1,6-bisP + H_2O → fructose-6-P + P_i

J   Fructose-6-P → glucose-6-P

K   Glucose-6-P + H_2O → glucose + P_i

   a. C, E, J, K
   b. A, B, E, K
   c. A, C, E, I
   d. A, B, I, K
   e. B, C, E, I

703. The different substrates of gluconeogenesis enter the pathway at different levels. In the following scheme, to which letter does correspond each one of the following compounds? (lactate, alanine, glycerol, propionyl-CoA)

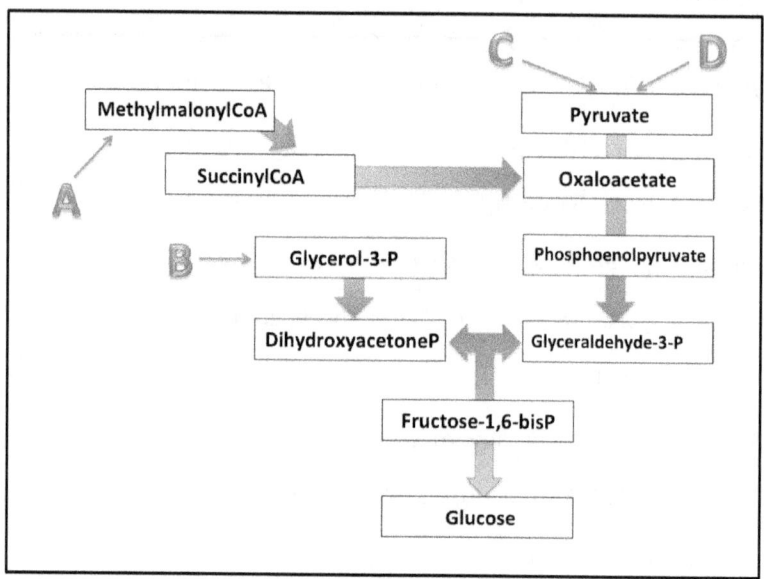

a. A=glycerol / B=lactate / C=propionyl-CoA / D= alanine
b. A=propionyl-CoA / B=lactate / C=glycerol / D= alanine
c. A=alanine / B=glycerol / C=propionyl-CoA / D= lactate
d. A=propionyl-CoA / B=glycerol / C=lactate / D= alanine
e. A=lactate / B=glycerol / C=propionyl-CoA / D= alanine

704. Which of the following compounds is an activator of gluconeogenesis?

a. fructose-2,6-bisP
b. AMP
c. acetylCoA
d. b and c
e. all are right

705. During intense exercise, glycogen muscular reserves are mobilized. Glucose is fast oxidized in an anaerobic way producing an excess of lactate, that is sent to blood. The destination of this lactate closes a metabolic cycle described by Carl and Gerti Cori in 1929, named Cori's cycle. Which is this destination of lactate?

a. It goes to brain, where it is converted into ketone bodies, that are metabolized, act as neurotransmitters and, after a few days, are metabolized to pyruvate, the to glucose, that returns to muscle to be oxidized or stored as glycogen.

b. It is again taken by the muscle, then converted into glucose and then waits to be oxidized through glycolysis, Krebs cycle and respiratory chain, as soon as the aerobic respiration may be possible.

c. goes to the liver, is converted into pyruvate, and then into glucose, that is sent to blood and taken by muscle to restore glycogen reserves.

d. goes to the liver, where it enters Krebs cycle and generates reducing power in form of NADH.

e. goes to the kidney, is converted into pyruvate, then into alanine or glutamine, by specific transaminases, and is used in the renal biosynthesis of amino acids.

706. In many ruminant animals, cellulose degradation produces large amounts of glucose that are to some extent fermented before being absorbed. This generates propanoate and lactate in large amounts. These compounds are incorporated into gluconeogenesis. How does lactate do this?

a. It is directly dehydrogenated to pyruvate.

b. It is directly converted into acetylCoA and, through Krebs cycle, produces pyruvate.

c. Is phosphorylated, generating phosphoenolpyruvate.

d. It is reduced forming glycerol, that produces dihydroxyacetone phosphate.

e. It is carboxylated producing oxaloacetate.

707. Glutamine is degraded within renal cortex, by the following reaction...

$$\text{glutamine} + H_2O \rightarrow \text{glutamate} + NH_3$$

...producing ammonia, that is used in urine pH regulation. The produced glutamate can be gluconeogenic substrate in these cells. How does this compound enter gluconeogenesis?

a. By the action of glutamate dehydrogenase, it is converted into lactate and ammonia, generating reducing power (NADH).

b. It is converted into α-ketoglutarate, generating ammonia and reducing power (NADH). The α-ketoglutarate turns into oxaloacetate through Krebs cycle.

c. It is converted into α-ketoglutarate, generating ammonia and consuming ATP. The α-ketoglutarate turns into oxaloacetate through Krebs cycle.

d. It is converted into succinylCoA, that turns into oxaloacetate by Krebs cycle.

e. It is decarboxylated by forming pyruvate, that by the action of cytosolic PEPCK turns into phosphoenolpyruvate.

Biosynthesis of other sugars and glycosylation of proteins

708. In the synthesis of lactose within mammary glands of mammals participate, among other, the following molecules...

    a. ATP, UTP, β-D-galactose, β-D-glucose and β-D-galactose-1-P
    b. UTP, UDP-galactose, β-D-glucose and β-D-galactose-1-P
    c. ATP, β-D-glucose and β-D-glucose-1-P
    d. a and b are true
    e. a and c are true

709. Penicillin...

    a. inhibits gluconeogenesis in bacteria at phosphofructokinase-II (PFK2) level
    b. inhibits the assembly of the pieces that give rise to the structure of peptidoglycan in bacterial wall.
    c. degrades O-glycosidic bonds between N-acetylglucosamine and N-acetyl muramic acid of bacterial wall, thus degrading the structure of peptidoglycan.
    d. inhibits the enzyme responsible for anchoring lipoteichoic acids to bacterial membrane
    e. inhibits Na^+/K^+ of bacterial wall, thus avoiding the generation of ATP by electrostatic gradient

710. Glucosamine-6-phosphate is an aminosugar precursor of most of the aminosugars in the body. From which precursors is it generated?

    a. fructose-6-P and glutamine
    b. glucose and ammonia
    c. glucose-6-P and ammonia
    d. glucose-6-phosphate and asparagine
    e. glucose-1-phosphate and ammonia

711. Sialic acid (N-acetyl muramic acid) is generated in a series of chain-reactions starting from UDP-N-acetylglucosamine. Within these reactions, there are two phosphorylated high-energy compounds that energetically contribute to some steps. Which are?

    a. ATP and GTP
    b. ATP and PEP
    c. ATP and creatinine-P
    d. ATP and fructose-6-P
    e. ATP and glucose-6-P

712. Proteins can undergo N-glycosylation in some residues. Which is the most common form?

a. An N-acetylglucosamine residue bound to the amide nitrogen of any peptide bond
b. An N-acetylglucosamine residue bound to the amide nitrogen of a lysine
c. An N-acetylglucosamine residue bound to the amide nitrogen of a glutamine
d. An N-acetylglucosamine residue bound to the amide nitrogen of a asparagine
e. An N-acetylglucosamine residue bound to the amide nitrogen of a arginine

713. Proteins can undergo O-glycosylation in some residues. Which is the most common form?

a. An N-acetylgalactosamine residue bound to a residue of valine or histidine
b. An N-acetylgalactosamine residue bound to a residue of tryptophan or tyrosine
c. An N-acetylgalactosamine residue bound to a residue of alanine or glutamine
d. An N-acetylgalactosamine residue bound to a residue of glycine or alanine
e. An N-acetylgalactosamine residue bound to a residue of serine or threonine

714. Molecular basis of the different blood types of the ABO system is based on the nature of some pentasaccharides bound to erythrocyte surface proteins. Which is the difference between A and B antigens?

a. a galactose present in A is absent in B
b. a galactose present in A is substituted by a glucose in B
c. a sialic acid present in A is changed by an N-acetylgalactosamine in B
d. an N-acetylgalactosamine present in A is substituted by a galactose in B
e. a fructose present in A is substituted by a glucose in B

715. Molecular basis for different blood types in the ABO system is based on the nature of some oligosaccharides bound to erythrocyte surface proteins. Which of the following assertions concerning oligosaccharides is TRUE?

a. they are O-glycosylations in which the following sugars are involved: fucose, galactose, N-acetylgalactosamine and sialic acid
b. they are O-glycosylations in which the following sugars are involved: glucose and galactose
c. they are N-glycosylations in which the following sugars are involved: N-acetylgalactosamine and sialic acid
d. they are N-glycosylations in which the following sugars are involved: N-acetylgalactosamine, N-acetylglucosamine, glucose and sialic acid
e. they are O-glycosylations in which the following sugars are involved: fucose, fructose and sialic acid

716. During the biosynthesis of blood antigens of ABO group, some monosaccharides (in particular N-acetylgalactosamine, sialic acid, galactose and fucose) are attached to a protein erythrocyte surface, forming a tetrasaccharide on which a final monosaccharide can be added. In this context, which of the following assertions is TRUE?

a. In people of 0 group, no more monosaccharides are added. The proteins remain only with this tetrasaccharide.
b. In people of A group, a glycosyltransferase that uses UDP-N-acetyl galactosamine as substrate adds it forming a pentasaccharide.
c. In people of B group, a galactosyltransferase that uses UDP-galactose as substrate adds it forming a pentasaccharide.
d. b and c are true
e. all are true

717. The synthesis of the oligosaccharides bound to proteins by nitrogen is very different to that of the ones bound by oxygen. Which of the following assertions, on N-linked oligosaccharides, is TRUE?

a. First of all, the oligosaccharide polymerizes without any support and later is added to the protein.
b. The oligosaccharide polymerizes on a mineral basis and, afterwards is added to the protein.
c. Oligosaccharide assembly is formed on an intermediate linked to lipids.
d. Oligosaccharide assembly is formed directly on the protein.
e. Directly, a monosaccharide binds to an asparagine residue, to this monosaccharide, as a chain reaction, other residues (mainly mannose) are added to form longer chains.

718. Most of the known oligosaccharides N-linked to proteins have a common structure. Which is it?

a. They organise from an N-acetylgalactosamine bound to an asparagine residue of the protein.
b. They organise around a dimer of N-acetylglucosamine and mannose bound to an asparagine residue of the protein.
c. They organise around a trimer of two mannoses and a glucose, bound to an asparagine residue of the protein.
d. They organise around a tetramer of two N-acetylglucosamines and two galactoses, bound to an asparagine residue of the protein.
e. They organise around a pentasaccharide with three mannoses and two N-acetylglucosamines, bound to an asparagine residue of the protein.

719. The synthesis of the oligosaccharides bound to proteins by nitrogen is very different of that of the ones bound by oxygen. Which of the following assertions, on N-linked oligosaccharides, is TRUE?

a. The oligosaccharide polymerizes on an steroid molecule and, afterwards, is added to the protein.
b. The oligosaccharide polymerizes on a dolichol phosphate molecule and, afterwards, is added to the protein.
c. The oligosaccharide polymerizes on a inositol triphosphate molecule and, afterwards, is added to the protein.
d. The oligosaccharide polymerizes on a gluthatione molecule and, afterwards, is added to the protein.
e. The oligosaccharide polymerizes on a pantothenic acid molecule and, afterwards, is added to the protein.

720. Most os the oligosaccharides bound to proteins by asparagine (N-linked) organise by following three structural patterns: complex structure, hybrid or high mannose. Besides, they assemble binding to a lipid derivative. Which of the following assertions, in this context, is FALSE?

a. The structural core is assembled linked to an isopreneid lipid called dolichol phosphate.
b. The binding with dolichol generally involves a glucose residue of the oligosaccharide.
c. Dolichol is made by using the same route that produces cholesterol and isopreneid compounds.
d. Dolichol is phosphorylated by a kinase that uses CTP.
e. Dolichol phosphate has only a phosphate group in its structure.

721. Most os the oligosaccharides bound to proteins by asparagine (N-linked) organise by following three structural patterns: complex structure, hybrid or high mannose. Which of the following assertions, in this context, is FALSE?

a. In high mannose structure, mannose residues (almost exclusively) are added to the main pentasaccharide.
b. In complex structure, N-acetylglucosamine, sialic acid, fucose and galactose residues are added in different proportions to the main pentasaccharide.
c. In hybrid structure, N-acetylglucosamine, sialic acid, fucose, mannose and galactose residues are added in different proportions to the main pentasaccharide.
d. Complex structure does not usually involve the addition of more mannose residues to the main pentasaccharide.
e. In high mannose structure, the oligosaccharide binds to asparagine directly by mannose, not involving any N-acetylglucosamine residue present in the main pentasaccharide.

722. The first step of the addition of sugars to proteins (biosynthesis of glycoproteins) is the binding of an oligosaccharide to a lipid, to be later attached to the protein. Where does this first step occur?

a. In the Golgi apparatus
b. In the endoplasmic reticulum
c. In the cell nucleus
d. In mitochondria
e. Outside the cell

723. The antibiotic tunicamycin inhibits the enzyme that catalyzes the binding between dolichol and UDP-N-acetylglucosamine. What effect does this drug have on cell physiology?

a. It blocks the addition of O-linked sugars to proteins
b. It blocks the addition of N-linked sugars to proteins
c. Inhibits electronic mitochondrial transport chain
d. Inhibits the synthesis of membrane glycophospholipids
e. It blocks dolichol β-oxidation

Lipid metabolism

General questions

724. How many ATPs are produced in the complete oxidation of palmitic acid (16C) through β-oxidation followed by Krebs cycle, electron transport chain and oxidative phosphorylation?
   a. 16
   b. 36
   c. 38
   d. 80
   e. 108

725. How many ATPs are needed to activate a fatty acid (transform it into acyl-CoA) to enter the β-oxidation process?
   a. 0
   b. 1
   c. 2
   d. 3
   e. 4

726. How many $FADH_2$ are produced in the complete oxidation of acid (16C) by β-oxidation?
   a. 1
   b. 7
   c. 8
   d. 15
   e. 16

727. How many NADH are produced in the complete oxidation of palmitic acid (16C) by β-oxidation?
   a. 1
   b. 7
   c. 8
   d. 15
   e. 16

728. How many AcetylCoA are produced in the complete oxidation of palmitic acid (16C) by β-oxidation?
   a. 2
   b. 4
   c. 8
   d. 16
   e. 32

Digestion, absortion and transport of lipids

729. Which of the following lipoproteins is the main way of transport for cholesterol from peripheral tissues to the liver, for its posterior metabolism or excretion?

a. chylomicrons
b. VLDL
c. IDL
d. LDL
e. HDL

730. Pancreatic lipase...

a. functions in an optimal way in the water-oil interface
b. needs to be bound to colipase to function
c. fragments triglycerides generating mainly 2-monoacylglycerides and fatty acids
d. a and b are right
e. all are right

731. Chylomicrons transport lipids mainly...

a. from intestine to tisuues
b. from lymphatic system to liver
c. from white adipose tissue to liver
d. from brown adipose tissue to liver
e. from brown adipose tissue to white adipose tissue, and vice versa

732. Chylomicrons are lipoproteins with roughly this chemical composition...

a. triglycerides (40-50%), phospholipids (10-20%), cholesterol (10-20%) and proteins (10-20%)
b. triglycerides (80-90%), phospholipids (5-10%), cholesterol (1-3%) and proteins (1-2%)
c. triglycerides (40-50%), phospholipids (30-40%), cholesterol (5-10%) and proteins (1-2%)
d. triglycerides (40-50%), phospholipids (5-10%), cholesterol (30-40%) and proteins (1-2%)
e. triglycerides (50-60%), phospholipids (10-20%), cholesterol (1-2%) and proteins (10-20%)

733. Chylomicrons are mainly produced...

a. in the liver
b. in duodenum epithelial cells
c. in B lymphocytes
d. in pancreas Langerhans cells
e. in the cells of renal medulla

734. Which of the following lipoproteins is the main way of transport of the triglycerides produced in the liver to the peripheral tissues?

a. chylomicrons
b. VLDL
c. IDL
d. LDL
e. HDL

735. Pancreatic lipase...

a. ...catalyzes the hydrolysis of triglycerides in positions 3 and 1, generating sequentially 1,2-diacylglycerols and 2-acylglycerols
b. ...catalyzes the hydrolysis of triglycerides in positions 2 and 3, generating sequentially 1,3-diacylglycerols and 1-acylglycerols
c. ...catalyzes the hydrolysis of triglycerides in positions 1 and 3, generating sequentially 2,3-diacylglycerols and 2-acylglycerols
d. ...catalyzes the hydrolysis of triglycerides in positions 3 and 2, generating sequentially 1,2-diacylglycerols and 1-acylglycerols
e. ...catalyzes the hydrolysis of triglycerides in positions 2 and 1, generating sequentially 1,3-diacylglycerols and 3-acylglycerols

736. The VLDL produced by the liver...

a. contain fats, cholesterol, cholesterol esters, apoprotein B100, apoprotein C1 and apoprotein E
b. when circulating in blood, take apoprotein C2 from HDL
c. when circulating in blood, take apoprotein E from HDL
d. a and c are right
e. all are right

737. Fat emulsions in the intestine...

a. ... are favoured by the presence of bile salts
b. ...are favoured by the action of pancreatic lipase that, when hydrolysing triglycerides, generates soap molecules, constituted by a fatty acid and a cation (Na^+ or K^+)
c. ...favour the action of pancreatic lipase that, as being soluble, can hydrolyse only the triglycerides that are in the fat-water interphase
d. ...increase the interaction surface between fats and water, thus favouring the action of digestive enzymes
e. All the previous answers are true.

738. So that triglycerides contained in chylomicrons and VLDL may be hydrolysed, a protein of these particles must activate lipoprotein lipase. Which is this protein?

a. apoprotein B-100
b. apoprotein C-I
c. apoprotein C-II
d. apoprotein C-III
e. apoprotein D

739. The following table shows the percentage (of total dry mass) corresponding to each one of the components of a series of lipoproteins.

	A	B	C	D	E
Proteins	15	50	2	23	9
Triglycerides	31	5	85	6	53
Free cholesterol	7	5	3	7	8
Cholesterol esters	23	12	4	43	10
Phospholipids	22	28	6	21	20

Indicate to which type of lipoproteins do the letters A, B, C and D correspond.

a. A=IDL, B=HDL, C=QM, D=LDL, E=VLDL
b. A=HDL, B=LDL, C=IDL, D=VLDL, E=QM
c. A=QM, B=VLDL, C=IDL, D=LDL, E=HDL
d. A=QM, B=VLDL, C=LDL, D=IDL, E=HDL
e. A=VLDL, B=LDL, C=QM, D=HDL, E=IDL

740. In the capillaries of peripheral tissues, lipoprotein lipase acts on the triglycerides of chylomicrons and of VLDL generating soluble fatty acids and 2-monoacylglycerides. Some of the released fatty acids are absorbed near the reaction, but other are transported by blood to more distant places. Which is the main transport way?

a. associated to serum albumin
b. dissolved in plasma
c. aggregated forming micelles with monovalent cations
d. associated to cholesterol esters, forming large insoluble aggregates
e. within macrophages, that previously have phagocyted them

741. Which of the following proteins is minority, or even nonexistent, in chylomicrons?

a. apoprotein A-I
b. apoprotein C-I
c. apoprotein C-III
d. apoprotein B-48
e. apoprotein E

742. The active site of pancreatic lipase contains a catalytic triad...

a. ...that resembles that used by hemoglobin fr the reversible binding of O_2
b. ...that allows a catalytic mechanism analogous to the formation of disulfide bridges by thioreductases
c. ...that resembles that of serin-proteases
d. ...that allows a mechanism analogous to pyruvate hydrolysis in pyruvate dehydrogenase complex
e. ...very similar to the one that catalyzes the addition of a phosphate to glucose in the enzyme hexokinase

743. What is the action made by lipoprotein lipase (LPL) when it acts on VLDL?

a. It attracts macrophages, thus accelerating the digestion of VLDL
b. It allows the recruitment of fats by the tissues
c. It allows the complete oxidation of acetylCoA produced in the β-oxidation
d. It oxidizes the fatty acids forming volatile aldehydes and allowing the emulsion of these particles
e. It reduces the fatty acids forming volatile aldehydes and allowing the emulsion of these particles

744. Phospholipase A_2...

a. ...hydrolyzes the fatty acid bound to the C2 of phospholipids, generating lisophospholipids
b. ...hydrolyzes the fatty acid bound to the C1 of phospholipids, generating lisophospholipids
c. ...hydrolyzes the fatty acids bound to the C1 and the C2 of phospholipids, generating phosphoglycerate and soaps of sodium or potassium
d. a and c are true
e. b and c are true

745. Phosphatidylcholine...

a. ...is a phospholipid secreted in the bile that helps in fat digestion
b. ...is a phospholipase A_2 substrate
c. ...is modified by the enzyme LCAT forming lisophosphatidylcholine
d. only a and b are true
e. a, b and c are true

746. In which organ/tissue is cholesterol mainly produced?

a. liver
b. kidney
c. heart
d. white adipose tissue
e. brown adipose tissue

747. Among the following lipoproteins, which is the main transport form of lipids from the intestine to peripheral tissues?
a. chylomicrons
b. VLDL
c. IDL
d. LDL
e. HDL

748. Which of the following proteins is almost exclusively found in chylomicrons?
a. apoprotein A-I
b. apoprotein C-I
c. apoprotein C-III
d. apoprotein B-48
e. apoprotein E

749. Bile salts...

a. facilitate the emulsion of fats, and so, their digestion
b. allow that fats may form aggregates, thus facilitating their excretion
c. hydrolyse fats generating glycerol and free fatty acids
d. hydrolyse fats generating 2-monoacylglycerides and free fatty acids
e. hydrolyse fats generating diacylglycerides and free fatty acids

750. When an intense activity of triglyceride hydrolysis (catalysed by lipoprotein lipase) takes place on chylomicrons, these particles are degradated to some particles with much more abundance of proteins. How do we name these particles?

a. chylomicron remains
b. VLDL
c. IDL
d. LDL
e. liposomes

751. Which of the following proteins is minority, or even nonexistent, in chylomicrons?

a. apoprotein A-I
b. apoprotein C-I
c. apoprotein C-III
d. apoprotein B-48
e. apoprotein B-100

752. Which of the following protein lists is most typical of HDL?

a. apoprotein B-100 ; apoprotein C-I ; apoprotein C-II ; apoprotein C-III ; apoprotein D
b. apoprotein A-I ; apoprotein A-II ; apoprotein C-I ; apoprotein C-II ; apoprotein C-III ; apoprotein D ; apoprotein E
c. apoprotein A-I ; apoprotein A-II ; apoprotein B-48 ; apoprotein C-I ; apoprotein C-II ; apoprotein C-III ;
d. apoprotein B-100 ; apoprotein C-I ; apoprotein C-II ; apoprotein C-III ; apoprotein E
e. apoprotein B-100

753. Which of the following lipoproteins is the main mode of transport of cholesterol towards peripheral tissues?

a. chylomicrons
b. VLDL
c. IDL
d. LDL
e. HDL

754. Which of the following protein lists is most typical of LDL?

a. apoprotein B-100 ; apoprotein C-I ; apoprotein C-II ; apoprotein C-III ; apoprotein D
b. apoprotein A-I ; apoprotein A-II ; apoprotein C-I ; apoprotein C-II ; apoprotein C-III ; apoprotein D ; apoprotein E
c. apoprotein A-I ; apoprotein A-II ; apoprotein B-48 ; apoprotein C-I ; apoprotein C-II ; apoprotein C-III ;
d. apoprotein B-100 ; apoprotein C-I ; apoprotein C-II ; apoprotein C-III ; apoprotein E
e. apoprotein B-100

755. Which of the following protein lists is most typical of VLDL?

a. apoprotein B-100 ; apoprotein C-I ; apoprotein C-II ; apoprotein C-III ; apoprotein D

b. apoprotein A-I ; apoprotein A-II ; apoprotein C-I ; apoprotein C-II ; apoprotein C-III ; apoprotein D ; apoprotein E

c. apoprotein A-I ; apoprotein A-II ; apoprotein B-48 ; apoprotein C-I ; apoprotein C-II ; apoprotein C-III ;

d. apoprotein B-100 ; apoprotein C-I ; apoprotein C-II ; apoprotein C-III ; apoprotein E

e. apoprotein B-100

756. Which of the following protein lists is most typical of chylomicrons?

a. apoprotein B-100 ; apoprotein C-I ; apoprotein C-II ; apoprotein C-III ; apoprotein D

b. apoprotein A-I ; apoprotein A-II ; apoprotein C-I ; apoprotein C-II ; apoprotein C-III ; apoprotein D ; apoprotein E

c. apoprotein A-I ; apoprotein A-II ; apoprotein B-48 ; apoprotein C-I ; apoprotein C-II ; apoprotein C-III ;

d. apoprotein B-100 ; apoprotein C-I ; apoprotein C-II ; apoprotein C-III ; apoprotein E

e. apoprotein B-100

757. When an intense activity of triglyceride hydrolysis (catalysed by lipoprotein lipase) takes place on VLDL, these particles are degradated to some particles with much more abundance of proteins. How do we name these particles?

a. VLDL remains
b. chylomicrons
c. IDL
d. LDL
e. liposomes

Oxidation of fatty acids

758. In which place of the cell does fatty acids β-oxidation occur?

   a. In the mitochondria
   b. In the lysosomes
   c. In Golgi apparatus
   d. In the endoplasmic reticulum
   e. In the ribosomes

759. Which is the balanced chemical equation for palmitoyl-CoA (16C) complete β-oxidation?

   a. Palmitoyl-CoA + 7 CoA-SH + 7 FAD + 7 NAD^+ + 7 H_2O → 8 AcetylCoA + 7 $FADH_2$ + 7 NADH + 7 H^+
   b. Palmitoyl-CoA + 8 CoA-SH + 8 FAD + 8 NAD^+ + 8 H_2O → 8 AcetylCoA + 8 $FADH_2$ + 8 NADH + 8 H^+
   c. Palmitoyl-CoA + 7 CoA-SH + 7 FAD + 7 $NADP^+$ + 7 H_2O → 8 AcetylCoA + 7 $FADH_2$ + 7 NADPH + 7 H^+
   d. Palmitoyl-CoA + 8 CoA-SH + 8 FAD + 8 $NADP^+$ + 8 H_2O → 8 AcetylCoA + 8 $FADH_2$ + 8 NADPH + 8 H^+
   e. Palmitoyl-CoA + 7 CoA-SH + 16 NAD^+ → 8 AcetylCoA + 16 NADH + 16 H^+

760. At the beginning of 20ᵗʰ century (1904) a series of very complete experiments performed by a German chemist, by using the methyl → phenyl substitution as metabolic tracer and overtaking to the appearing of radioactive tracers, allow to dilucidate the pathway of fatty acids within eukaryotic cells. Who was this chemist?

   a. Lothar Andgewante
   b. Franz Knoop
   c. Feodor Lynen
   d. Adouls Diels-Alder
   e. Frederick Wittig

761. The following scheme represents the entry of 'activated' fatty acids (acyl-CoA) in mitochondria to start β-oxidation. To which proteins or compounds do the letters A, B, C, D, E and F correspond?

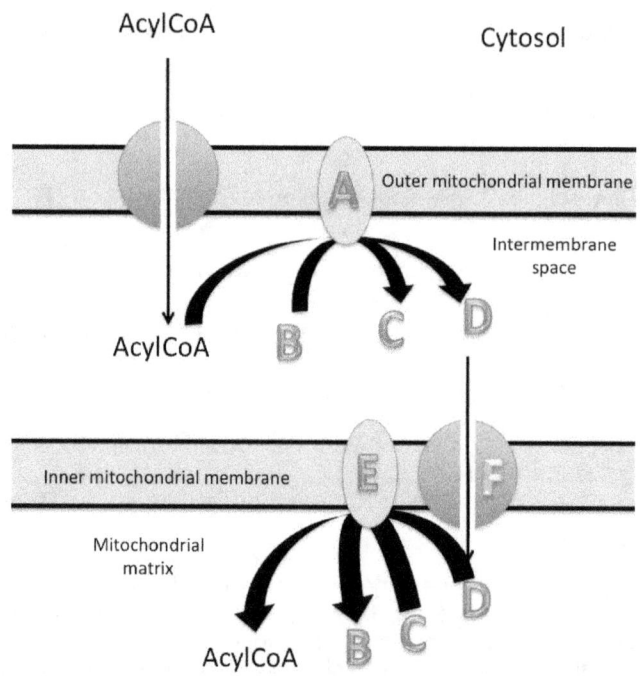

a. A=acyl-CoA kinase / B=ATP / C=ADP / D=phospho-acyl-CoA / E=acyl-CoA phosphatase / F=phospho-acyl-CoA transporter

b. A=acyl-CoA transporter / B=carnitine / C=CoA-SH / D=acylcarnitine / E=carnitine acyltransferase / F=acylcarnitine transporter

c. A=acyl-CoA kinase / B=ATP / C=ADP / D=phospho-acyl-CoA / E=phospho-acyl-CoA phosphatase / F=acylporine

d. A=carnitine acyltransferase I / B=carnitine / C=CoA-SH / D=acylcarnitine / E=carnitine acyltransferase II / F= acylcarnitine transporter

e. A=acyl-CoA dehydrogenase / B=NADPH / C=NADP+ / D= acyl-CoA carboxylate / E=acyl-CoA dehydrogenase / F=monocarboxylate transporter

762. The fatty acids present in cytosol, to be introduced into mitochondrial matrix, need to be 'activated' by a process in several steps outside the mitochondria. When it comes to this process, which of the following assertions is FALSE?

    a. fatty acids first bind an ATP molecule forming an adenylate of the fatty acid
    b. to the adenylate of the fatty acid, a carnitine is bound to form acyl carnitine
    c. carnitine is substituted by coenzyme A, to form an acyl-CoA
    d. acyl-CoA passes through external mitochondrial membrane by a transporter
    e. all are right

763. In the β-oxidation of fatty acids a series of cyclic steps are produced. In each one, the fatty acid reduces its length releasing a molecule of...

    a. formylCoA
    b. acetylCoA
    c. propionyl-CoA
    d. malonylCoA
    e. propanoate

764. Each cycle of β-oxidation is composed by four steps or reactions. In the first one of them, an acyl-CoA dehydrogenase catalyzes the following reaction...

    a. Acyl-S-CoA + NAD$^+$ → cis-Δ2-enoyl-S-CoA + NADH + H$^+$
    b. Acyl-S-CoA + E-FAD → trans-Δ2-enoyl-S-CoA + E-FADH$_2$
    c. Acyl-S-CoA + NAD$^+$ → trans-Δ2-enoyl-S-CoA + NADH + H$^+$
    d. Acyl-S-CoA + E-FAD → cis-Δ2-enoyl-S-CoA + E-FADH$_2$
    e. Acyl-S-CoA + E-FAD → trans-Δ3-enoyl-S-CoA + E-FADH$_2$

765. The following scheme is a simplification of the experiments performed, at the beginning of the 20th century (1904), by the German chemist Franz Knoop, that allowed to elucidate the nature of the pathway of fatty acids degradation in eukaryotic cells.

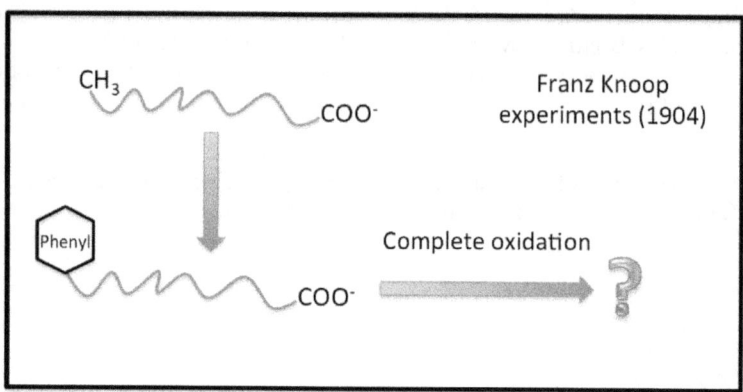

In them, the terminal methyl group of fatty acids is substituted by phenyl. Once the fatty acid has been completely degraded by biological oxidation, a different result was obtained depending on its number of carbons (even/odd). Which compound was obtained when oxidizing fatty acids with an odd number of carbons?

a. phenylalanine
b. phenylacetic acid
c. benzoic acid
d. phenylpropanoic acid
e. phenylbutyric acid

766. The FAD-dependent oxidation of acyl-CoA (first step of each β-oxidation cycle) is followed by...

a. a decarboxylation of acyl-CoA
b. a hydration
c. a NAD⁺-dependent dehydrogenation
d. other FAD-dependent dehydrogenation
e. a NADP⁺-dependent dehydrogenation

767. In hepatic mitochondria, acetylCoA produced in β-oxidation can have an alternative destination, instead of entering Krebs cycle. It is ketogenesis. This route begins with the generation of acetoacetylCoA, by using the thiolase reaction in an inverse way. This acetoacetylCoA is converted into HMG-CoA by HMGCoA synthase and, specifically in the liver, HMG-CoA lyase converts it into acetoacetate and acetylCoA. How does this route continue towards the production of ketone bodies and, in particular, acetone?

a. AcetylCoA enters Krebs cycle to form citrate, that is broken forming propanoate, that is decarboxylated to acetone.
b. AcetylCoA enters Krebs cycle to form citrate, that is broken forming three molecules of acetic acid, that are reduced to form acetone.
c. AcetylCoA loses CoA-SH, directly generating acetone.
d. Acetoacetate is reduced to β-hydroxybutyrate or, in a lower proportion, is decarboxylated to acetone.
e. Acetoacetate is decarboxylated forming acetic acid, that is then reduced to acetone.

768. Each β-oxidation cycle is constituted by four steps or reactions. In the first one, an acyl-CoA dehydrogenase catalyzes an acyl-CoA oxidation (formation of a *trans* double bond). Afterwards, enoylCoA hydratase catalyzes the following reaction...

a. trans-Δ2-enoyl-S-CoA + H_2O → L-3-hydroxyacyl-S-CoA + CO_2
b. trans-Δ2-enoyl-S-CoA + H_2O → D-2-hydroxyacyl-S-CoA + acetylCoA
c. trans-Δ2-enoyl-S-CoA + H_2O → D-2-hydroxyacyl + acetylCoA
d. trans-Δ2-enoyl-S-CoA + H_2O → L-3-hydroxyacyl-S-CoA
e. trans-Δ2-enoyl-S-CoA + E-FAD → L-3-hydroxyacyl-S-CoA + E-$FADH_2$

769. The complete oxidation of a cytosolic palmitic acid (16 C) to CO_2 and water, after suffering the corresponding activation to palmitoyl-CoA, complete β-oxidation and complete oxidation complete of acetylCoA and reduced coenzymes generated (NADH and $FADH_2$) through Krebs cycle, electron transport chain and oxidative phosphorylation, has a net energetic yield of...

a. 37 ATPs
b. 38 ATPs
c. 57 ATPs
d. 129 ATPs
e. 136 ATPs

770. The following scheme is a simplification of the experiments performed, at the beginning of the 20th century (1904), by the German chemist Franz Knoop, that allowed to elucidate the nature of the pathway of fatty acids degradation in eukaryotic cells.

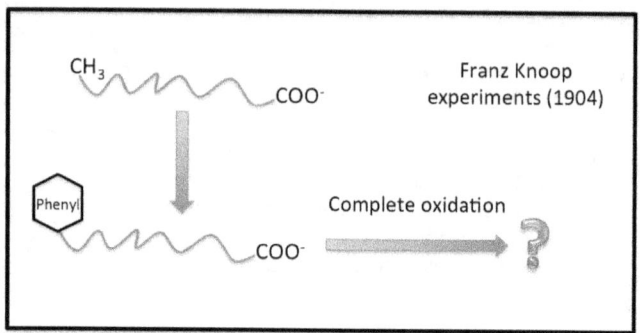

In them, the terminal methyl group of fatty acids is substituted by phenyl. Once the fatty acid has been completely degraded by biological oxidation, a different result was obtained depending on its number of carbons (even/odd). Which compound was obtained when oxidizing fatty acids with an even number of carbons?

a. phenylalanine
b. phenylacetic acid
c. benzoic acid
d. phenylpropanoic acid
e. phenylbutyric acid

771. The complete oxidation of a cytosolic palmitic acid (16 C) by β-oxidation generates...

a. 3 FADH$_2$
b. 4 FADH$_2$
c. 5 FADH$_2$
d. 6 FADH$_2$
e. 7 FADH$_2$

772. Each β-oxidation cycle is made up of four steps or reactions. In the firs one, an acyl-CoA dehydrogenase catalyzes the following reaction...

$$Acyl-S-CoA + E-FAD \rightarrow trans-\Delta2-enoyl-S-CoA + E-FADH_2$$

Which of the following assertions on this reaction is FALSE?

a. the electrons of $FADH_2$ are transferred to a shuttle protein called ETFP (electron transfer flavoprotein)
b. the electrons of ETFP are directly transferred to cytochrome a_3, in the mitochondrial electron transport chain, by the action of the enzyme EFT-Q oxidoreductase
c. the chemical mechanism of dehydrogenase is an elimination reaction type E2
d. the acyl-CoA dehydrogenase is constituted by four monomers, each one having a bound $FAD/FADH_2$
e. the mechanism initiates with the deprotonation of the α carbon of the fatty acid, by the action of a glutamic acid of acyl-CoA dehydrogenase

773. Each β-oxidation cycle is made up of four steps or reactions. In the firs one, an acyl-CoA dehydrogenase catalyzes the oxidation of an acyl-CoA (*trans* double bond formation). Afterwards, enoylCoA hydratase catalyzes the following reaction:

$$trans-\Delta2-enoyl-S-CoA + H_2O \rightarrow L-3-hydroxyacyl-S-CoA$$

Then, 3-hydroxyacyl-CoA dehydrogenase acts. Which of the following reactions is the one catalysed by this enzyme?

a. L-3-hydroxyacyl-S-CoA $\rightarrow$ 3-cetoacyl-S-CoA + H_2O
b. L-3-hydroxyacyl-S-CoA + NAD^+ $\rightarrow$ 3-cetoacyl-S-CoA + NADH + H^+
c. L-3-hydroxyacyl-S-CoA + $NADP^+$ $\rightarrow$ 3-cetoacyl-S-CoA + NADPH + H^+
d. L-3-hydroxyacyl-S-CoA + $NADP^+$ $\rightarrow$ 2-cetoacyl-S-CoA + NADPH + H^+
e. L-3-hydroxyacyl-S-CoA + E-FAD $\rightarrow$ 3-cetoacyl-S-CoA + E-FADH$_2$

774. Within the peroxisomes of eukaryotic cells, a unique β-oxidation of fatty acids takes place, defined by the following characteristic...

a. The final product in the route is the malonylCoA, that normally comes from gluconeogenesis
b. The electrons taken by acyl-CoA dehydrogenase, instead of passing to coenzyme Q within mitochondrial electron transport chain, are transferred to O_2, that is reduced to H_2O_2, that is finally eliminated by catalase
c. The first attack occurs on α-carbon, displacing a carbon all the later reactions. So, each two cycle turns, a CO_2 and an acetylCoA are produced
d. The first attack occurs on α-carbon, displacing a carbon all the later reactions. So, each cycle turn, a CO_2 and an acetylCoA are produced
e. The produced acetylCoA crystallize forming oxalate crystals, that can be observed by phase contrast microscopy

775. In conditions of high [acetylCoA] and low [oxaloacetate], the acetylCoA produced in β-oxidation can enter in an inverse way in thiolase reaction, forming acetoacetyl-CoA. Which is the most common destination, among the ones mentioned, of this compound?

a. To be transformed into HMG-CoA and initiate the synthesis of cholesterol
b. To be transformed into α-ketoglutarate and enter Krebs cycle
c. To be transformed into succinil-CoA and enter Krebs cycle
d. To be transformed into acetate through acetic fermentation, thus obtaining reducing power (NADH)
e. To nourish the biosynthesis of acyl-CoAs by means of lipogenesis

776. In each β-oxidation cycle, we distinguish four steps or reactions. The last one of them starts from 3-cetoacyl-CoA as sustrate, and is catalyzed β-cetothiolase. Which is the chemical equation for this reaction?

a. 3-cetoacyl-CoA → fatty acid + acetylCoA
b. 3-cetoacyl-CoA + NAD^+ → acyl-CoA + NADH + H^+
c. 3-cetoacyl-CoA + $NADP^+$ → acyl-CoA + NADPH + H^+
d. 3-cetoacyl-CoA + CoA-SH → acyl-CoA + acetylCoA
e. 3-cetoacyl-CoA + H_2O → acetylCoA + CO_2

777. The complete oxidation of a cytosolic palmitic acid (16 C) by β-oxidation generates...

a. 3 NADH
b. 4 NADH
c. 5 NADH
d. 6 NADH
e. 7 NADH

778. In hepatic mitochondria, the acetylCoA produced in β-oxidation can have an alternative destination, instead of entering Krebs cycle. It is ketogenesis. Which circumstances do trigger this route?

a. a high concentration of acetylCoA and oxaloacetate
b. a low concentration of de acetylCoA and oxaloacetate
c. a high concentration of acetylCoA and a low concentration of oxaloacetate
d. a low concentration of acetylCoA and a high concentration of oxaloacetate
e. none of the previous oprions does involve a significative activation of this route

Lipogenesis

779. The adipocytes of white adipose tissue have a very low activity of glycerol kinase. From where do they mainly obtain the glycerol-3-phosphate used in the synthesis of new triglycerides?

a. From β-oxidation
b. From glycolysis
c. From photosynthesis
d. From Cori's cycle
e. From Krebs cycle

780. The synthesis of palmitate in adipocytes basically lies in cycles of stepped addition of compounds of ____ carbons to the forming fatty acid.

a. 1
b. 2
c. 3
d. 4
e. 5

781. Which of the following equation does correspond to the complete biosynthesis of a palmitate molecule (16 C) from acetylCoA?

a. 8 acetylCoA + 8 ATP + 16 NADPH + 16 H$^+$ → palmitate + 16 NADP$^+$ + 8 CoA-SH + 8 H$_2$O + 8 ADP + 8 P$_i$
b. 8 acetylCoA + 7 ATP + 14 NADPH + 13 H$^+$ → palmitate + 14 NADP$^+$ + 8 CoA-SH + 6 H$_2$O + 7 ADP + 7 P$_i$
c. 8 acetylCoA + 8 ATP → palmitate + 8 CoA-SH + 6 H$_2$O + 8 ADP + 8 P$_i$
d. 8 acetylCoA + 8 ATP → palmitate + 8 ADP + 8 P$_i$
e. 8 acetylCoA + 16 NADPH + 16 H$^+$ → palmitate + 16 NADP$^+$ + 8 CoA-SH + 8 H$_2$O

782. The synthesis of palmitate in adipocytes begins with the action of acetyl-CoA carboxylase, that combines acetylCoA and bicarbonate para dar lugar a...

a. malonyl-CoA
b. HMGCoA
c. succinylCoA
d. 2-β-OH-butyrylCoA
e. 3-β-OH-butyrylCoA

783. The enzyme that limits the velocity of lipogenesis is...

a. HGMCoA reductase
b. AcetylCoa carboxylase
c. Malonyl-CoA-ACP transacylase
d. AcetylCoA-ACP transacylase
e. Enoyl-ACP reductase

784. The synthesis de fatty acids desde acetylCoA incluye numerosos pasos intermedios en los que los fatty acids en formación se encuentran unidos covalentemente a un compuesto químico. ¿Cuál es?

a. CoA-SH
b. carnitine
c. ACP (protein transportadora del acilo)
d. FMN
e. HMGCoA-SH

785. Synthesis of malonylCoA from acetylCoA spends, for each produced malonylCoA,...

a. 1 ATP
b. 1 GTP
c. 1 NADH
d. 1 NADPH
e. 1 $FADH_2$

786. By one of the following mechanisms, long-chain acyl-CoA act on acetylCoA carboxylase, inhibiting lipogenesis. Which is this mechanism?

a. They activate the depolymerisation of the acetylCoA carboxylase filaments
b. They indirectly cause the massive phosphorylation of acetylCoA synthase
c. They indirectly cause the massive dephosphorylation of acetylCoA synthase
d. They stimulate the addition of certain N-glycosylations on specific asparagine residues of acetylCoA carboxylase
e. They bind to acetylCoA carboxylase forming insoluble aggregates

787. The synthesis of malonyl-CoA from acetylCoA is catalysed by acetylCoA carboxylase. This enzyme has a cofactor bound by the amino ε group of a lysine. Which cofactor is it?

a. TPP
b. ascorbic acid
c. FMN
d. biotin
e. pantothenic acid

788. The following scheme indicates the steps that go from acetylCoA to the synthesis of a fatty acid precursor of 4 carbons (butyryl-ACP). Which compounds are represented by A, B, C, D and E letters?

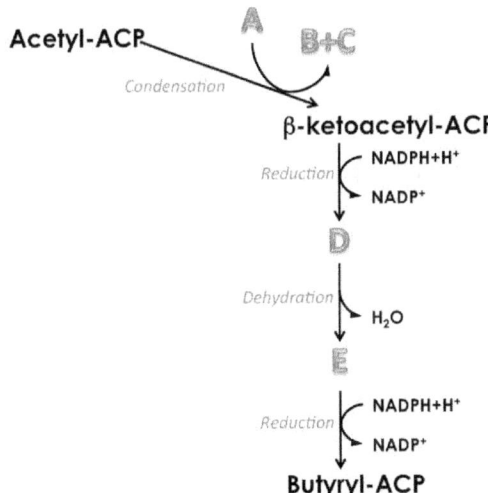

a. HMGCoA / malonyl-CoA / CO_2 / β-hydroxyacyl-ACP / trans-Δ3-enoyl-ACP
b. malonyl-CoA / acetate / CO_2 / D-3-hydroxyacyl-ACP / cis-Δ2-enoyl-ACP
c. malonyl-CoA / acetate / CO_2 / cis-Δ3-hydroxyacyl-ACP / cis-Δ3-enoyl-ACP
d. malonyl-CoA / acetate / CO_2 / β-hydroxyacyl-ACP / trans-Δ3-enoyl-ACP
e. malonyl-CoA / ACP / CO_2 / D-3-hydroxyacyl-ACP / trans-Δ2-enoyl-ACP

789. In a reaction catalysed by acyl-CoA desaturase, the activated form of stearic acid (18:0) turns into the activated form of oleic acid (18:1ΔA9), one of the most frequent monounsaturated fatty acids in animals. Which is the equation of the complete reaction?

a. stearoylCoA + NADPH + H^+ + O_2 → oleylCoA + $NADP^+$

b. stearoylCoA + NADPH + H^+ + O_2 → oleylCoA + $NADP^+$ + 2 CO_2

c. stearoylCoA + NADH + H^+ + O_2 → oleylCoA + NAD^+ + 2 H_2O

d. stearoylCoA + NADPH + H^+ + O_2 → oleylCoA + $NADP^+$ + 2 H_2O

e. stearoylCoA + NADH + H^+ → oleylCoA + NAD^+

Biosynthesis of steroids, terpenes, porphyrins and eicosanoids

790. Cholesterol and other steroids derive from the cyclation of a 30-carbon containing polyterpene named...

a. isoprene
b. cyclopentanoperhydrophenanthrene
c. polystyrene
d. mevalonate
e. squalene

791. Which of the following steps does pertain to the process of cholesterol synthesis?

a. The conversion of 2-carbon residues (acetate o acetylCoA) into 6-carbon compounds (mevalonic acid)
b. The transformation of 6 units of mevalonic acid (6 C) into 6 units of isopentenyl pyrophosphate (5 C)
c. The combination of 6 units of isopentenyl pyrophosphate (5 C) to produce a molecule of squalene (30 C)
d. The cyclation of squalene and the loss of three carbons, to lead to cholesterol
e. All are right

792. Which of the following values may be right if we consider that they refer to the amount of bile acids daily secreted to intestine lumen by an average man?

a. 2 g
b. 25 g
c. 500 mg
d. 500 g
e. 2 mg

793. Cholesterol synthesis begins with the production of mevalonate from acetylCoA, where does this take place?

a. Within mitochondria
b. Within cytosol
c. Within endoplasmic reticulum
d. b and c are right
e. All are right

794. Cholesterol synthesis begins with the production of mevalonate from acetylCoA, as represented in the following diagram. What do A, B, C and D letters stand for?

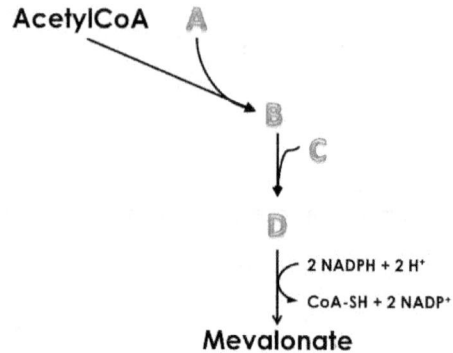

a. acetylCoA / acetoacetylCoA / acetylCoA / 3-OH-3-methylglutaryl-CoA
b. CO_2 / propionyl-CoA / acetylCoA / 3-OH-3-methylglutaryl-CoA
c. CO_2 / malonyl-CoA / acetylCoA / 2-OH-2-methylglutaryl-CoA
d. acetylCoA / acetoacetylCoA / malonyl-CoA / 2-OH-2-methylglutaryl-CoA
e. acetate / malonyl-CoA / acetylCoA / 2-OH-2-methylglutaryl-CoA

795. The transformation of β-carotene into vitamina A_1 (all-*trans*-retinol) involves...

a. A dioxygenase and a reductase
b. NADPH coenzymes, that are oxidized to $NADP^+$
c. Chemical energy in form of ATP
d. a and b are true
e. All are true

796. Cholesterol synthesis begins with the production of mevalonate from acetylCoA. A characteristic enzyme of steroid biosynthesis participates in this process. Which is?

a. HMGCoA reductase
b. Mevalonate synthase
c. AcetoacetylCoA decarboxylase
d. AcetoacetylCoA dehydrogenase
e. AcetylCoA reductase

797. HMGCoA reductase...

a. inhibits when phosphorylated by AMP-activated protein kinase
b. is activated (at a transcriptional level) by farnesol, a mevalonate derivative
c. inhibits (at a transcriptional level) when cholesterol concentration decreases
d. a and c are right
e. all are right

798. This is the synthesis of bile salts from cholesterol. What do A, B and C letters stand for?

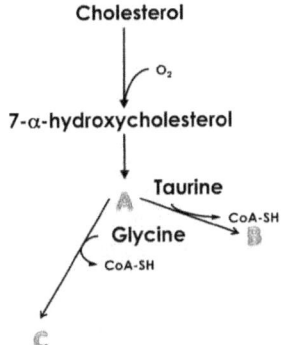

a. cholylCoA / taurocholate / glycocholate
b. HMGCoA / taurilCoA / glycochole
c. lanosterylCoA / lanosterol / squalene
d. squalenylCoA / taurocholate / glycocholate
e. malonyl-CoA / taurocholate /glycocholate

799. Which of the following values may be right if we consider that they refer to the amount of bile acids daily secreted to intestine lumen by an average man and not recovered by enterohepatic circulation?

a. 2 g
b. 25 g
c. 500 mg
d. 500 g
e. 2 mg

800. The following diagram shows in a simplified way the synthesis of several steroid hormones. To which compounds do A, B, C and D letters correspond?

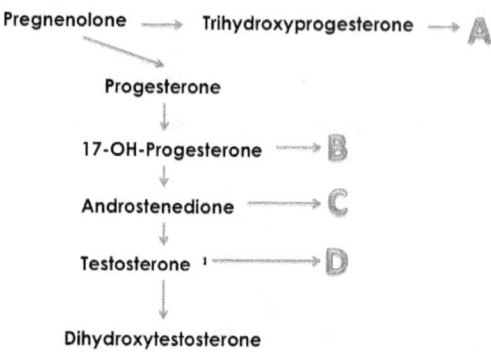

a. aldosterone / cortisol / estrone / estradiol
b. estradiol / aldosterone / estrone / cortisol
c. estradiol / aldosterone / cortisol / estrone
d. cortisol / estradiol / aldosterone / estrone
e. aldosterone / estradiol / estrone / cortisol

801. Bilirrubin...

a. is a catabolic product of heme group
b. is a product of urea cycle
c. is an intermediate of Krebs cycle
d. is a precursor of hepatic gluconeogenesis
e. is a product of cholesterol degradation

802. Hemo-oxygenase catalyzes the transformation of heme group into biliverdin. Which the equation of this chemical reaction?

a. heme + O_2 + NADPH + H^+ → biliverdin + Fe^{3+} + $NADP^+$ + H_2O + CO_2
b. heme + NADH + H^+ → biliverdin + NAD^+
c. heme + O_2 → biliverdin + Fe^{3+} + H_2O
d. heme + O_2 → biliverdin + Fe^{3+} + CO_2
e. heme + O_2 → biliverdin + CO_2

803. Biliverdin reductase catalyzes the transformation of biliverdin into bilirrubin, as shown in the following picture. Which compounds do A and B letters stand for?

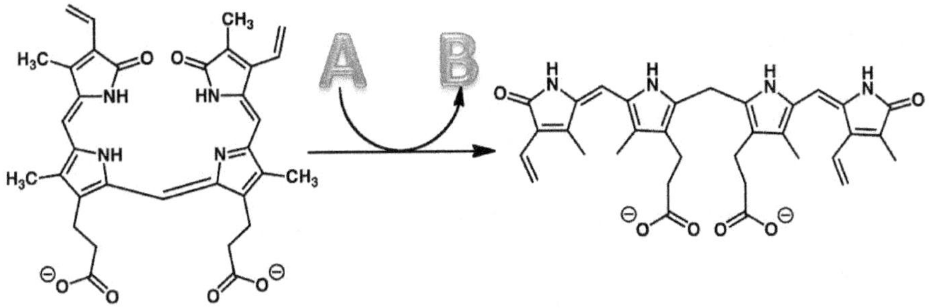

a. A=H_2O; B=nothing
b. A=(CoA-SH + NADH + H^+); B=NAD^+
c. A=(NADH + H^+); B=NAD^+
d. A=(NADPH + H^+); B=$NADP^+$
e. A=(NAD^+); B=NADH + H^+

804. An student has written some reactions presumably involved in heme group hepatic biosynthesis. Which of them is an error?

a. 4 porphobilinogen (PBG) → uroporphyrinogen-III + 4 NH_4^+ + H_2O
b. 2 succinylCoA + 2 glycine → 2 aminolevulinato + 2 CoA + 2 CO_2
c. uroporphyrinogen-III + 4 CO_2 → coporphyrinogen-III
d. coporphyrinogen-III + O_2 → 2 CO_2 + protoporphyrinogen-IX
e. protoporphyrinogen-IX → protoporphyrin-IX + 6 H^+

805. Porphyrins are produced from an amino acid (_____) and a Krebs cycle intermediate (_____).

a. glycine / succinylCoA
b. alanine / α-ketoglutarate
c. lysine / α-ketoglutarate
d. serine / succinate
e. serine / fumarate

Endocrine control of lipid and sugar metabolism

806. Which of the following assertions on the effects of an insulin rise in liver is FALSE?

a. It activates hepatic glycogenesis
b. It activates lipogenesis
c. It activates gluconeogenesis
d. a and b
e. b and c

807. Which of the following is not an effect of glucagon?

a. It activates hepatic glycogenesis
b. It activates lipolysis in white adipose tissue
c. It activates hepatic glycogenolysis
d. a and b
e. b and c

808. Which of the following is NOT an effect of insulin?

a. It stimulates glucose intake by the muscle
b. It stimulates glucose intake by white adipose tissue
c. It stimulates lipogenesis in white adipose tissue
d. It stimulates glycogenesis in skeletal striated muscle
e. It stimulates hepatic gluconeogenesis

809. Adrenalin...

a. inhibits glycogenolysis in skeletal striated muscle
b. activates lipolysis in white adipose tissue
c. activates glycogenesis in liver
d. inhibits gluconeogenesis in liver
e. b and d are right

810. In the muscle...

a. insulin stimulates glucose intake
b. adrenalin stimulates glycogenolysis
c. insulinstimulates glycogenesis
d. b and c are right
e. all are right

811. In white adipose tissue...

a. adrenalin inhibits lipolysis
b. glucagon inhibits lipolysis
c. insulin blocks glucose intake
d. insulin activates lipogenesis
e. a and d are right

812. Which of the following assertions is FALSE?

a. Insulin causes dephosphorylation and resulting activation of pyruvate dehydrogenase
b. Insulin accelerates the flux of glucose across plasma membrane
c. Insulin favours the synthesis of triglycerides
d. Insulin stimulates lipogenesis (production of fatty acids from acetylCoA)
e. Insulin stimulates glycogenolysis

813. In the liver...

a. Glycogenesis is activated by insulin and inhibited by glucagon and adrenalin
b. Insulin activates lipogenesis
c. Gluconeogenesis is activated by insulin and inhibited by adrenalin
d. Glycogenolysis is inhibited by glucagon
e. a and b are right

Amino acid metabolism

814. Which of the following chemical formulas does correspond to urea?

a. $(CH_3)_2CO$
b. $(NH_2)_2CO$
c. $(CH_3)NH$
d. $NH_2-NH-CH_3$
e. $CH_3-CO_2-NH_2$

815. Urea cycle...

a. ...was firstly described by James Watson and Francis Crick (1932)
b. ... was firstly described by Thomas Morgan and Theodosius Dobzhansky (1932)
c. ... was firstly described by por John Urey and Stanley Miller (1932)
d. ... was firstly described by por Max Perutz and Severo Ochoa (1932)
e. ... was firstly described by por Hans Krebs and Kurt Henseleit (1932)

816. Urea cycle...

a. ...in mammals mainly takes place in the liver and, to a lower extent, in the kidney
b. ...in mammals mainly takes place in the brain and, to a lower extent, in the walls of digestive system
c. ...in mammals mainly takes place in erythrocytes and, to a lower extent, in the smooth muscle
d. ...in mammals mainly takes place in skeletal muscle and, to a lower extent, in the smooth muscle
e. ...in mammals mainly takes place in the kidney and, to a lower extent, in the smooth muscle

817. If the velocity of urea cycle becomes lower than usually...

a. ...blood glucose level will increase
b. ...the levels of adrenocorticotropic hormone will increase
c. ...the amount of nitrogenated products in the blood, specially ammonia, will increase
d. ...blood lactate and pyruvate levels will increase
e. ...the amount of phenolic compounds in blood will increase in the liver and in the blood

818. In the renal cortex, ammonia is produced to regulate urine pH. Which is the main amino acid, quantitatively, from which this ammonia is generated?

a. arginine
b. glycine
c. asparagine
d. glutamine
e. alanine

819. Large amounts of nitrogen are sent from muscle an other tissues to the liver, through the blood. In this travel, nitrogen can not be as NH_4^+, since it would modify too much several physicochemical parameters of the blood. In form of which copounds is it mainly transported?

a. glutamate and glutamine
b. arginine and glutamate
c. glutamine and α-ketoglutarate
d. alanine and urea
e. glutamine and alanine

820. The nitrogen present in muscle in the form of NH_4^+ is transported to the liver in form of alanine. How is it incorporated to this amino acid?

a. In a process catalysed by alanine transaminase, ammonia is added to pyruvate forming glutamine. By other transaminase, this glutamine generates alanine, regenerating the initial pyruvate.
b. In a reaction catalysed by glutamate dehydrogenase, ammonia is added to α-ketoglutarate to produce glutamate. This glutamate later joins pyruvate, in a process catalysed by a transaminase, to form alanine and regenerate the α-ketoglutarate used at the beginning.
c. By the action of glutamate dehydrogenase, ammonia joins α-ketoglutarate to produce 2-aminosuccinate. This compound later joins glutamate, in a process catalysed by a transaminase, to form alanine and regenerate the α-ketoglutarate used at the beginning.
d. It joins bicarbonate ion to form carbamoyl phosphate and, by urea cyce, form urea, that is carboxylated to alanine.
e. In a reaction catalysed by alanine transaminase, ammonia is added to lactate, directly forming alanine.

821. In most of tissues, except the muscle, the majoritary form of transporting nitrogen, that is in form of NH_4^+, is by incorporating it to glutamine by means of glutamine synthetase. Which is the reaction catalysed by this enzyme?

a. Glutamate + NH_4^+ + ATP → Glutamine + ADP + P_i + H_2O
b. Aspartate + NH_4^+ → Glutamine + H_2O
c. Pyruvate + NH_4^+ + ATP → Glutamine + ADP + P_i
d. Pyruvate + NH_4^+ + ATP → Glutamine + ADP + P_i + H_2O
e. Pyruvate + NH_4^+ + NADH + H^+ → Glutamine + NAD^+ + H_2O

822. The incorporation of ammonia to glutamate, forming glutamine that will be transported to the liver, is a process catalysed by glutamine synthetase in the majority of the tissues, that entails an energetic consumption of...

a. 1 ATP for each incorporated ammonia
b. 1 NADH for each incorporated ammonia
c. 1 $FADH_2$ for each incorporated ammonia
d. 2 ATPs for each incorporated ammonia
e. 1 GTP for each incorporated ammonia

823. Which of the following assertions is FALSE?

a. Hepatic alanine transaminase works mainly joining α-ketoglutarate and alanine to form glutamate and pyruvate
b. The pyruvate generated by hepatic alanine transaminase is mainly directed to gluconeogenesis, to produce glucose that will be sent, in its majority, to muscle
c. Hepatic glutamate dehydrogenase works mainly joining α-ketoglutarate and ammonia to form glutamate
d. Muscular alanine transaminase works mainly joining glutamate and pyruvate to form alanine and α-ketoglutarate
e. Ammonia is transported in form of alanine from the muscle to the liver, where it is released to enter urea cycle

824. The transaminase GPT catalyzes the following reaction...

a. aspartate + α-ketoglutarate → oxaloacetate + glutamate
b. aspartate + oxaloacetate → α-ketoglutarate + glutamate
c. alanine + glutamate → α-ketoglutarate + pyruvate
d. alanine + pyruvate → α-ketoglutarate + glutamate
e. alanine + α-ketoglutarate → pyruvate + glutamate

825. The transaminase GOT catalyzes the following reaction...

a. aspartate + α-ketoglutarate → oxaloacetate + glutamate
b. aspartate + oxaloacetate → α-ketoglutarate + glutamate
c. alanine + glutamate → α-ketoglutarate + pyruvate
d. alanine + pyruvate → α-ketoglutarate + glutamate
e. alanine + α-ketoglutarate → pyruvate + glutamate

826. In which organ is the urea mainly produced?

a. liver
b. kidney
c. heart
d. thyroid
e. bone marrow

827. Urea in human body is made by urea cycle. Quantitatively, this process has the most intensity in a particular organ, which is?

a. Kidney
b. Brain
c. Bone marrow
d. Spleen
e. Liver

828. Which of the following assertions is FALSE?

a. Ammonotelic animals are those that excrete nitrogen in form of ammonia
b. Most of of land animals are ureotelic, that is, they excrete nitrogen as urea
c. Most of aves and reptiles are uricotelic, that is, they excrete nitrogen as uric acid
d. The five steps of urea cycle take place within hepatocyte mitochondria
e. Urea cycle was firstly described, by the 1930s century, by Hans Krebs and his student Kurt Henseleit

829. Which of the following assertions is FALSE?

a. A 10-15% of the energy resulting from amino acid oxidation is lost in urea production. To compensate these losses, some ruminants add urea to the rumen and use it in the synthesis of new amino acids.

b. To transport free ammonia to liver, the majority of tissues transform glutamate into glutamine, that travels through blood to liver and there is again transformed into glutamate, transferring ammonia to urea cycle.

c. The tissue that processes the highest amount of nitrogen introducing it into urea cycle is the liver.

d. Muscular alanine transaminase works mainly joining glutamate and pyruvate to produce alanine and α-ketoglutarate

e. a and d are false

830. The ammonia present within mitochondrial matrix of hepatocytes is mixed with the CO_2 coming from cell respiration giving rise, thanks to ATP consumption, to carbamoyl phosphate. This reaction is catalysed by carbamoyl phosphate synthetase. Which of the following compounds is an allosteric activator of this enzyme?

a. acetylCoA

b. serotonin

c. N-acetyl muramic acid

d. AMP_c

e. N-acetyl glutamate

831. Inside the mitochondria, in the urea cycle, the carbamoyl phosphate and the ornithine form a nitrogenated compound that exits to cytosol. Which is?

a. Urea

b. Argino-succinate

c. Citruline

d. Fumarate

e. Carbamine

832. Which of the following reactions does not pertain to urea cycle?

a. Carbamoyl phosphate + ornithine → citruline + P_i
b. Argino-succinate → fumarate + arginine
c. Arginine + H_2O → Ornithine + Urea
d. Citruline + Aspartate + ATP → Argino-succinate + AMP + PP_i
e. None

833. How many high-energy phosphates does the synthesis of a molecule of urea, through one turn of urea cycle, require?

a. 1
b. 2
c. 3
d. 4
e. 5

834. Where is required, within urea cycle, the hydrolysis of ATP?

a. In the formation of carbamoyl phosphate
b. In the formation of urea
c. In the formation of argino-succinate
d. a and c are right
e. All are right

835. Which equation does describe the global matter flux of urea cycle?

a. $2\,NH_4^+ + HCO_3^- + 3\,ATP + H_2O$ → urea + $2\,ADP + AMP + 4\,P_i + 5\,H^+$
b. $2\,NH_4^+ + HCO_3^-$ → urea + $5\,H^+$
c. $NH_4^+ + HCO_3^- + 3\,ATP + H_2O$ → urea + $2\,ADP + AMP + 4\,P_i + H^+$
d. $2\,NH_4^+ + HNO_3^- + 2\,ATP + H_2O$ → urea + $ADP + AMP + 3\,P_i + 3\,H^+$
e. $2\,NH_4^+ + HNO_3^- + 2\,ATP + H_2O$ → urea + $2\,ADP + 2\,P_i + 3\,H^+$

836. Which of the following assertions on protein degradation is FALSE?

a. Ubiquitin, in an ATP-dependent reaction, condensates some of its glycine residues with lysine residues of the target protein.
b. Ubiquitin-labelled proteins are driven towards the proteasome and degraded.
c. The amino acid residues most given to oxidation by Fe^{2+} and OH^- are glutamate and aspartate.
d. Short-life proteins (mean lifetime lower than 2 hours) tend to have one or more regions (of about 12 to 60 amino acids) specially rich in proline, glutamate, serine and threonine.
e. The mean lifetime of an intracellular protein is statistically very correlated to the nature of the amino acid found at an N-terminal position. It has been seen that, if it is tyrosine, tryptophan or phenylalanine, protein lifetime is shorter.

837. The enzyme L-amino acid oxidase, found in the liver, catalyzes...

a. The elimination of the amino group in β position of an amino acid, converting it into an oxo group.
b. The elimination of the amino group in α position of an amino acid, converting it onto an oxo group.
c. The elimination of the amino group in α position of an amino acid, leaving a methylene in that position.
d. The elimination of the amino group in β position of an amino acid, leaving a methylene in that position.
e. The elimination of the amino group in β position of an amino acid, leaving an hydroxyle in that position.

838. The enzyme L-amino acid oxidase, found in liver and kidney, catalyzes an amino acid oxidation. To which coenzyme does it transfer the electrons produced in this oxidation?

a. FAD^+
b. NAD^+
c. coenzyme A
d. $NADP^+$
e. FMN

839. This diagram represents the steps of Krebs-Henseleit urea cycle. What do A, B, C, D E, F, G, H, I, J, K and L letters stand for?

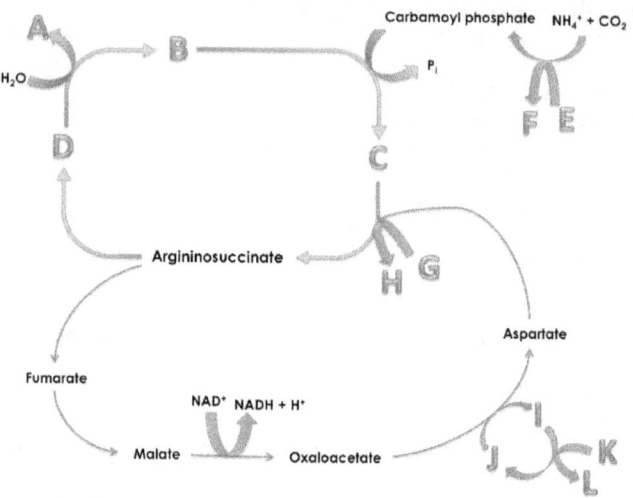

a. urea / ornithine / citruline / arginine / 2 ATP / 2 ADP + P_i / ATP / AMP + PP_i / α-ketoglutarate / glutamate / NH_4^+ + NADH + H^+ / H_2O + NAD^+

b. urea / citruline / ornithine / arginine / ATP / ADP + P_i / ATP / ADP + P_i / α-ketoglutarate / glutamate / NH_4^+ + NADH + H^+ / H_2O + NAD^+

c. urea / ornithine / citruline / arginine / ATP / 2 ADP + P_i / ATP / ADP + P_i / α-ketoglutarate / glutamate / NH_4^+ + NADH + H^+ / H_2O + NAD^+

d. urea / citruline / arginine / ornithine / 2 ATP / 2 ADP + P_i / ATP / AMP + PP_i / α-ketoglutarate / glutamate / NH_4^+ + NADH + H^+ / H_2O + NAD^+

e. urea / citruline / arginine / ornithine / ATP / ADP + P_i / ATP / ADP + P_i / glutamate / α-ketoglutarate / NH_4^+ + NAD^+ / H_2O + NADH + H^+

840. Phenylketonuria is a genetic disease characterized by the disability of the patient to transform phenylalanine into tyrosine. It is usually caused by a deficiency in the enzyme phenylalanine hydrolase or the enzyme tetrahydrobiopterin reductase. What is observed in patients of this pathology?

a. They have a paler skin, given that tyrosine is a precursor of melanin synthesis.
b. They present an increase of phenylalanine levels in urine.
c. It is necessary to enrich their diet with tyrosine
d. a, b and c are right
e. Only b and c are right

841. Which of the following amino acids is essential in humans?

a. alanine
b. asparagine
c. proline
d. glutamic acid
e. histidine

842. An important proportion of carbon flux between the proteins of peripheral tissues and liver is made through the release of some amino acids to blood, that are finally recruited by liver and nourish the processes of gluconeogenesis and urea cycle. Which amino acids are?

a. glycine and valine
b. serine and threonine
c. alanine and glutamine
d. glutamate and aspartate
e. proline and histidine

843. Which of the following lists does contain exclusively amino acids that are essential for humans?

a. FVTWIMHRLK
b. QWI
c. FSNMRLHKTV
d. DESNMRLHKTV
e. FSDNMRLHKEV

844. Which of the following assertions on amino acid biosynthesis in humans is FALSE?

a. Cysteine tends to be considered as a non-essential amino acid since it can be produced from serine, but to a certain extent it is essential, since the sulfur that it incorporates comes from methionine, that must be included in diet.
b. Phenylalanine is an essential amino acid and, starting from it, we can produce tyrosine.
c. Alanine is not an essential amino acid. It can be directly made from pyruvate, through transamination.
d. Serine is not an essential amino acid. It can be directly produced from 3-phosphoglycerate, through transamination.
e. There are biosynthetic pathways that synthesize the heterocyclic lateral chain of tryptophan in humans. Although this synthesis is specific of some renal cortex regions, it can be considered as a non-essential amino acid.

845. Alanine is made from pyruvate, through a transamination reaction coupled to other transamination towards the reverse direction. Which is the second coupled reaction?

a. glutamate → α-ketoglutarate
b. valine → α-ketoisovalerate
c. cysteine → α-ketocistinate
d. a and b
e. all are true

846. There is an amino acid that can be made from the ornithine produced in the urea cycle, and it provides quantities enough of this amino acid for an adult. However, for growing people, this rate of synthesis is not sufficient, so it tends to be considered as an essential amino acid. Which is it?

a. phenylalanine
b. tryptophan
c. methionine
d. arginine
e. lysine

847. The pathway for the biosynthesis of histidine (in E.coli) begins with a precursor named...

a. ribose-5-phosphate
b. 5-phosphoribosyl pyrophosphate
c. citidin monophosphate
d. inulin-triphosphate
e. inositol-triphosphate

848. _____ is directly synthesized from _____, although it requires the sulphur derived from _____.

a. cysteine / serine / methionine
b. cysteine / alanine / methionine
c. methionine / serine / cysteine
d. methionine / alanine / cysteine
e. methionine / threonine / cysteine

849. There is an amino acid that must be included in diet as a precursor of tyrosine. Which is?

a. proline
b. tryptophan
c. phenylalanine
d. histidine
e. arginine

850. Phenylalanine _____ is a critical step in the metabolism of such amino acid, being crucial for its transformation into tyrosine, thyroid hormones or catecholamines.

a. acetylation
b. hydroxylation
c. hydrogenation
d. transamination
e. phosphorylation

851. Lysine is synthesized from _____ through _____ pathway

a. pyruvate / Creutzfeldt's
b. alanine / pentose phosphate
c. aspartate / diaminopimelate
d. arginine / hepatic transaminases
e. arginine / chorismate

852. The synthesis of the amino acids glutamate, glutamine, proline and arginine is mainly performed from a Krebs cycle intermediate. Which is?

a. citrate
b. α-ketoglutarate
c. succinate
d. fumarate
e. oxaloacetate

853. The synthesis of serine passes through the following intermediates ...

a. 3-phosphoglycerate / phosphohydroxylpyruvate / phosphoserine / serine
b. dihydroxyacetonephosphate / glyceraldehyde-3-phosphate / serine
c. 1,3-bisP-glycerate / 2-phosphoglycerate / phosphoenolpyruvate /serine
d. erythrose-4-phosphate / erythrose-1,4-bisP / glutamine phosphate /serine
e. glutamine phosphate / glutamine /serine

854. The synthesis de phenylalanine, tyrosine and tryptophan have in common the formation of a previous intermediate called _____, that is generated from _____ and _____.

a. chorismate / phosphoenolpyruvate / erythrose-4-phosphate
b. benzoic acid / phenol / carbonic acid
c. 2-metil-butadiene / carbamoyl phosphate / bicarbonate
d. salicylic acid / 3-phosphoglycerate / acetylCoA
e. histidine / glutamine / benzoic acid

855. This diagram represents two intermediate steps in the biosynthesis of an amino acid, which is?

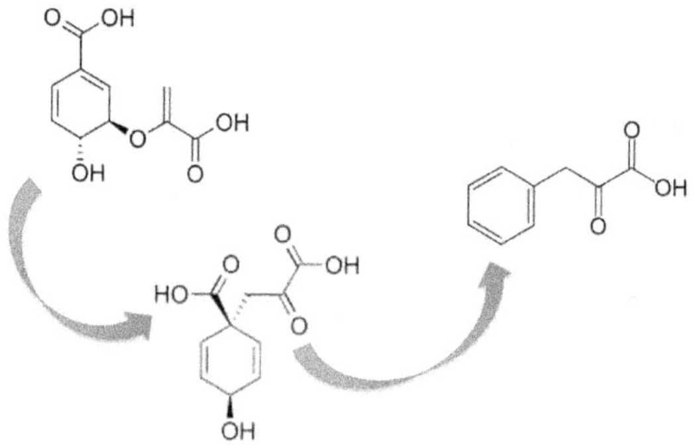

a. methionine
b. phenylalanine
c. glycine
d. valine
e. lysine

856. Aspartokinase is an enzyme that catalyzes the phosphorylation of aspartic acid, that is a previous step for its conversion into other amino acids. Into which amino acids is usually aspartic acid transformed?

a. lysine
b. methionine
c. asparagine
d. a and c
e. all are true

857. The biosynthesis of an amino acid passes through a compound named chorismate. This compound is transformed into anthranilate by a enzyme that requires nitrogen provided by ammonia or glutamine. Finally we arrive to the mentioned amino acid. Which is?

a. histidine
b. tryptophan
c. lysine
d. glutamic acid
e. threonine

858. Methionine can be converted, by the action of an enzyme, into S-adenosyl-methionine (SAM). Which of the following is a usual role for SAM in biological systems?

a. It acts as methyl groups donor, associated to several enzymes.
b. It regulates blood pH, like gluthatione.
c. It is a thyroid hormone precursor.
d. It is a cofactor in the reaction of iodation of tyrosine to form thyroid hormones.
e. It acts as an energetic coin.

Nucleotide metabolism

859. The pathway of purine biosynthesis begins with ribose-5-P and ends in a compound named...

a. adenine
b. adenine monophosphate (AMP)
c. cyclic adenine monophosphate (AMPc)
d. guanine triphosphate (GTP)
e. inosine monophosphate (IMP)

860. In the pathway of purine synthesis, the enzyme ribose phosphate pyrophosphokinase adds a phosphate to ribose-5-P (coming from pentose phosphate pathway) generating...

a. 5-phosphoribosyl pyrophosphate (PRPP)
b. 1-phosphoribosyl pyrophosphate (PRPP)
c. ribose-1,5-bisP (RbP)
d. ribose-2,5-bisP (RbP)
e. ribose-3,5-bisP (RbP)

861. To synthesize a molecule of inosine monophosphate (IMP) from ribose-5-P we need...

a. 1 ATP molecule
b. 2 ATP molecules
c. 3 ATP molecules
d. 4 ATP molecules
e. 5 ATP molecules

862. Inosine monophosphate can be transformed into guanine monophosphate in two steps, passing through an intermediate named...

a. adenosine monophosphate (AMP)
b. diphosphate of guanidinium
c. guanosine triphosphate (GTP)
d. oxanosine monophosphate (OMP)
e. xanthine monophosphate (XMP)

863. In the pathway of purine synthesis, the enzyme amidophosphoribosyltransferase catalyzes the transformation of PRPP into 5-phosphoribosylamine, as is shown in the following diagram.

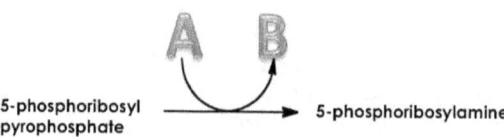

5-phosphoribosyl
pyrophosphate
——————————→ 5-phosphoribosylamine

What do A and B letters stand for?

    a. A=glutamine; B=(glutamate + PP$_i$)
    b. A=serine; B=(pyruvate + PP$_i$)
    c. A=glutamine; B=(glutamate)
    d. A=serine; B=(pyruvate)
    e. A=(serine + ATP); B=(pyruvate + AMP + PP$_i$)

864. Adenosine monophosphate can be converted into guanine monophosphate in two steps, passing through an intermediate called...

    a. adenyl diphosphate
    b. adenylsuccinate
    c. adenyl-CoA
    d. natrine monophosphate (NMP)
    e. xanthine monophosphate (XMP)

865. The conversion of IMP into adenyl-succinate, catalysed by adenyl-succinate synthetase, follows this reaction...

    a. IMP + glutamate + GTP → GDP + adenyl-succinate
    b. IMP + ATP → ADP + adenyl-succinate
    c. IMP + GTP → GDP + adenyl-succinate
    d. IMP + aspartate + GTP → GDP + adenyl-succinate
    e. IMP + glutamate + ATP → ADP + adenyl-succinate

866. Uric acid...

    a. ...y el ascorbic acid have a high antioxidant power.
    b. ...comes from the action of xanthine oxidase on the heterocycle xanthine.
    c. ...is the final product of purine metabolism in humans.
    d. b and c are true.
    e. todas son ciertas

867. The conversion from adenyl-succinate to AMP, catalysed by adenyl-succinate lyase, follows this chemical reaction...

a. adenyl-succinate + ATP → ADP + P$_i$ + AMP
b. adenyl-succinate + ATP → ADP + P$_i$ + succinate + AMP
c. adenyl-succinate + ATP → ADP + P$_i$ + succinylCoA + AMP
d. adenyl-succinate + ATP → ADP + P$_i$ + fumarate + AMP
e. adenyl-succinate → fumarate + AMP

868. The conversion from IMP to XMP, catalysed by IMP-dehydrogenase, follows this chemical reaction...

a. IMP → XMP
b. IMP + NAD$^+$ → XMP + NADH + H$^+$
c. IMP + H$_2$O + NAD$^+$ → XMP + NADH + H$^+$
d. IMP + NADH + H$^+$ → XMP + NAD$^+$
e. IMP + H$_2$O + NADH + H$^+$ → XMP + NAD$^+$

869. Which of the following assertions on uric acid metabolism is FALSE?

a. The majority of mammals (except for many primates) convert uric acid into allantoin.
b. The Dalmatian dogs cannot convert uric acid into allantoin, so they are among the few mammals that excrete uric acid, resembling in this aspect to humans.
c. Uric acid and ascorbic acid have a high antioxidant power. It is very likely that uric acid can play in non-primate mammals the role of vitamin C in humans.
d. Aves and reptiles directly excrete uric acid in solid form.
e. Copper activates xanthine oxidase and iron inhibits it. So, plasma levels of both metals (that vary with the age of individual) modulate the rate of uric acid production.

870. The conversion of XMP into GMP, catalysed by GMP-synthetase, follows this chemical reaction...

a. XMP + glutamine + ATP → GMP + glutamate + AMP
b. XMP + ATP → GMP + AMP
c. XMP + glutamine → GMP + glutamate
d. XMP + serine + ATP → GMP + pyruvate + AMP
e. XMP + serine → GMP + pyruvate

871. Purine base, to be degraded, are all transformed into _____, that afterwards is transformed into _____, that is the final product of amine catabolism in mammals.

a. inosine / inulin
b. inosine / xanthine
c. inosine / hypoxanthine
d. xantine / uric acid
e. inosine / uric acid

872. The precursor of all pyrimidine nucleotides in the cell is...

a. uridine monophosphate (UMP)
b. thymidine monophosphate (TMP)
c. 5-OH-thymidine monophosphate (5-OH-TMP)
d. cytidine monophosphate (UMP)
e. isocytidine monophosphate (IMP)

873. The following list of compounds indicate the intermediates that appear in the biosynthesis *de novo* of uridine monophosphate (UMP). Which is the right list?

a. fumarate / carbamoylphosphate / carbamoylaspartate / dihydroorotate / orotate / UMP
b. glutamine / carbamoylphosphate / orotate / TMP / UMP
c. methionine / carbamoylphosphate / 5-OH-pyridine / orotate / UMP
d. bicarbonate + glutamine / carbamoylphosphate / carbamoylaspartate / dihydroorotate / orotate / UMP
e. serotonin / aspartate / UMP

Metabolic diseases

874. The cystinuria...

a. is a disruption of kidney reabsorption mechanisms for dibasic amino acids.
b. is a disruption of the transamination of cystinate to synthesize cysteine.
c. is a disruption of cysteine catabolism.
d. is a disruption due to the deficiency of the enzyme that provides serine with sulphur to synthesize cysteine.
e. b and c are right.

875. Among the drugs for the treatment of type-II diabetes, we find sulfonylureas. What is their action mechanism?

a. They increase the capture of glucose by the tissues.
b. They increase the sensitivity of the tissues towards insulin.
c. They stimulate insulin secretion.
d. They decrease blood acidosis.
e. a and b are true.

876. Type-II diabetes mellitus is characterized by...

a. ...low blood levels of glucagon
b. ... low blood levels of glucose
c. ... low blood levels of hierro
d. ... low blood levels of adrenalin
e. ... low blood levels of insulin

877. Which of the following is a symptom of type I diabetes mellitus?

a. An increase in the total amount of urine (polyuria).
b. Excessive thirst (polydipsia)
c. Excessive hunger (polyphagia)
d. Dry mouth (xerostomia)
e. All are right

878. Various disruptions of lipid catabolism (deficiency in the transport of carnitine, deficiency in Acyl-CoA dehydrogenase and the Zellweger's syndrome) share a common sign. Which is?

a. presence of acetaldehyde in urine
b. presence of acetona in urine
c. presence of medium size chain fatty acids in urine
d. presence of insulin in urine
e. presence of acetylCoA in urine

879. The most frequent monogenic disease among those affecting glucidic metabolism, with an incidence of 1 of each 55000 births, is...

a. ...phenylketonuria
b. ...inability to metabolize galactose
c. ...deficiency of phosphofructokinase-II
d. ...deficiency of pyruvate carboxylase
e. ...Jacob's fever

880. The deficiency of arginosuccinate synthase causes...

a. phenylketonuria
b. cystinuria
c. succinaturia
d. galactosuria
e. citrulinuria

881. An excess of ammonia (NH_4^+) in the brain, specially at cerebellum and striatum, causes...

a. ...an important activation of NMDA (N-methyl-D-aspartate) receptors, increasing the concentration of GMP_c.
b. ...an activation of glutamate dehydrogenase in its function of α-ketoglutarate and ammonia into glutamate, slowing the speed of Krebs cycle and indirectly contributing to cell death.
c. ...an increase in the concentration of carbamoyl phosphate, that acts as a competitive antagonist of serotonin affecting to nervous function.
d. a and b are true.
e. All are true.

882. The majority of genetically caused galactosemia cases are produced by mutations in the gene of...

a. galactose-1-P uridylyltransferase
b. glycogen phosphorylase
c. lactase
d. phosphogalactomutasa
e. uridindiphosphate galactose-4-epimerase

883. There is a little frequent genetic disorder in which hepatic fructokinase is non-functional. Which symptom is most likely to accompany this disease...

a. An excess of fructose in urine (fructosuria).
b. Lowering of insulin blood levels.
c. Increase of glucagon blood levels.
d. a and c are true.
e. All are true.

884. What is the cause for type I diabetes?

a. The destruction of pancreas β cells.
b. Malignant ploriferation of cells within bone marrow.
c. The decrease of glucose blood levels.
d. The desensitization of the blood receptors for acidity located at aortic arch and carotid sinus.
e. The destruction of renal cortex parenchyma.

885. Which of the following is a symptom for type I diabetes mellitus?

a. Increase of the total urine amount (polyuria)
b. Weight loss.
c. Fatigue.
d. a and c are true.
e. All are true.

886. Among the most frequent complications of diabetes, we find diabetic neuropathy. Why is it produced?

a. Because aldose reductase generates much sorbitol, that enters the nervous system, thus inhibiting mioinositol entry within nervous cells. This indirectly affects to the behaviour of Na+/K+ ATPase in neurons and alters nervous conduction.

b. Because the excess of glucose is converted, thanks to a phosphoglucomutase, into allose. Allose transaminase produces two molecules of glutamate for each glucose that initiates the route. This great increase of the levels of glutamate (a neurotransmitter), strongly disrupts interneuranol communication.

c. Because of the excess of phosphorylated glucose, converted into galactose-6-P, and afterwards into galactose-1,6-bisP. A three-steps enzymatic pathway synthesizes serotonin from this reactive. This great increase of the levels of serotonin (a neurotransmitter), strongly disrupts interneuranol communication.

d. Because often the injected insulin generates local hypokalemia episodes in several locations within the brain, although it can also affect peripheral locations.

e. Since the excess of glucose, by a three-step enzymatic pathway, is converted into idose. An enzyme produces two molecules of GABA (γ-aminobutyric acid) for each glucose that initiates the route. This great increase of the levels of GABA (a neurotransmitter), strongly disrupts interneuranol communication.

887. A baby girl about 5 months old shows regular vomit episodes and she does not gain weight. Her behaviour markedly oscillates between periods of lethargy and excesive irritability. Electroencephalographies are abnormal and an unusually high ammonia concentration is detected in plasma (~550mg/dl when normal values are in the range 25-150 mg/dl). Glutamine concentration is also high in relation to basal values. Besides, a precursor of pyrimidine (orotate) is found in urine. Which of the following genetic disorders is likely to account for this clinical profile?

a. Type I diabetes mellitus.
b. Very reduced activity of hepatic ornithine transcarbamoylase.
c. Zellweger's syndrome (disability to correctly make peroxisomes).
d. Muscular citruline dehydrogenase is not functional.
e. Hepatic phosphofructokinase-I is not functional.

888. Which of the following signs, extracted from a blood test, may be indicative of homocystinuria?

a. High concentration of sodium and ammonia.
b. High concentration of carbamoyl phosphate.
c. High values of methionine and homocysteine dimers.
d. High concentration of hydrogen sulphide.
e. Unusually high (and very similar among them) values of cysteine and urea.

889. Phenylketonuria is a genetic disease characterized by the disability of the patient to transform phenylalanine into tyrosine. It is usually caused by a deficiency in the enzyme phenylalanine hydrolase or the enzyme tetrahydrobiopterin reductase. What is observed in patients of this pathology?

    a. They have a paler skin, given that tyrosine is a precursor of melanin synthesis.
    b. They present an increase of phenylalanine levels in urine.
    c. It is necessary to enrich their diet with tyrosine
    d. a, b and c are right
    e. Only b and c are right

890. Which of these signs is associated to maple syrup urine disease?

    a. Increase of the blood levels of the ketoacids corresponding to any amino acid.
    b. Increase of the blood levels of the ketoacids corresponding to branched-chain amino acid.
    c. Increase of the blood levels of aromatic amino acids in general.
    d. Increase of the blood levels of tryptophan.
    e. Increase of the blood levels of phenylalanine.

891. Among the drugs for the treatment of type II diabetes, we find biguanides (for example, metformin). What is its mechanism of action?

    a. They increase the capture of glucose by the tissues.
    b. They increase the sensitivity of the tissues towards insulin.
    c. They stimulate insulin secretion.
    d. They decrease blood acidosis.
    e. a and b are true.

892. La phenylketonuria...

    a. is the result of the deficiency in the enzyme phenylalanine phosphorylase
    b. is the result of the deficiency in the enzyme phenylalanine carboxykinase
    c. is the result of the deficiency in the enzyme phenylalanine transaminase
    d. is the result of the deficiency in the enzyme phenylalanine dehydrogenase
    e. is the result of the deficiency in the enzyme phenylalanine hydroxylase

893. Glycogen storage disease type I (von Gierke's disease) is caused by a deficiency in glucose-6-phosphatase, that generates...

a. ...an hypoglycemia during fasting that does not decrease when blood levels of insulin increase

b. ...an hypoglycemia during fasting that does not decrease when blood levels of glucagon or adrenalin increase

c. ...an hyperglycemia during the first 2-3 hours after lunch that does not decrease when increasing blood levels of insulin

d. ...una hyperglycemia during fasting that does not decrease when increasing blood levels of insulin

e. ...una hyperglycemia during fasting that does not decrease when increasing blood levels of glucagon or adrenalin

894. Which of the following assertions is FALSE?

a. Insulin increases potassium intake by cells.

b. The lack of insulin causes the release of potassium by cells, mainly in skeletal striated muscle.

c. The majority of patients hospitalized with a diabetic ketoacidosis show high levels of potassium in urine.

d. The majority of patients hospitalized with a diabetic ketoacidosis show high levels of potassium in blood.

e. The action of injecting insulin to patients with an acute diabetic ketoacidosis has an important risk of generating hypokalemia, that is very dangerous for cardiac muscle. So, potassium supplements are usually added to the treatments with insulin in this clinical profile.

895. Patients of phenylketonuria...

a. tend to have a very pale pigmentation

b. present a high amount of phenyl-lactate and phenylpyruvate in urine

c. present epilepsy with high frequency

d. a and b are true

e. all are true

896. Black urine disease (alkaptonuria)...

a. is caused by a deficiency in the enzyme that catalyzes the oxidation of homogentisic acid, an intermediate in the catabolism of phenylalanine and tyrosine
b. tends to derive in the accumulation of solid deposits in joints, resulting frequently in arthritis at the age of 30-40 years
c. is produced by a genetic defect in the pathway that goes from tyrosine to acetylCoA-fumarate within amino acid catabolism.
d. b and c are right
e. all are right

897. Among the drugs for the treatment of type II diabetes, we find thiazolidinediones (also known as glitazones). What is its mechanism of action?

a. They increase the capture of glucose by the tissues.
b. They increase the sensitivity of the tissues towards insulin.
c. They stimulate insulin secretion.
d. They decrease blood acidosis.
e. a and b are true.

898. Muscle glycogen phosphorylase deficiency (McArdle's disease) causes...

a. hypoglycemia
b. hyperglycemia
c. limitation for the patients to perform extreme physical exercise
d. a and c are right
e. b and c are right

899. Which of the following assertions on type I and type II diabetes mellitus is FALSE?

a. type I diabetes mellitus tends to be detected before the patient is 20 years old
b. type II diabetes mellitus tends to be detected after the patient is 40 years old
c. type II diabetes mellitus is caused by the degradation (probably as an autoimmunitary process) β cells of pancreas
d. type I diabetes mellitus shows an almost nonexistent insulin concentration in plasma
e. the positive response to antibodies against cells of Langerhans islets is indicative of type I diabetes mellitus

Carbohydrates biosynthesis in plants and bacteria. Photosynthesis.

General questions

900. Which of the following is the global equation of photosynthesis?

a. $3 CO_2 + 3 H_2O + light\ energy \rightarrow C_3H_6O_3 + 3 O_2$
b. $6 CO_2 + 6 H_2O + light\ energy \rightarrow C_6H_{12}O_6 + 6 O_2$
c. $6 O_2 + 6 H_2O + light\ energy \rightarrow C_6H_{12}O_6 + 6 CO_2$
d. $5 O_2 + 5 H_2O + light\ energy \rightarrow C_5H_{10}O_5 + 5 CO_2$
e. $5 CO_2 + 5 H_2O + light\ energy \rightarrow C_5H_{10}O_5 + 5 O_2$

901. The oxygen atoms present in the O_2 that is released by photosynthetic organisms, from which molecule(s) do come from?

a. From water
b. From water and CO_2
c. From CO_2
d. From glucose
e. From glucose and water

902. Chemosynthesis, by which purple sulphur bacteria fix atmospheric CO_2, is globally a redox process where CO_2 is reduced to organic matter and a reducing agent is oxidized. Which is this reducing agent?

a. H_2O
b. H_2S
c. HSO_3^-
d. H_2
e. Lactate

903. Photosynthesis of plants, green algae and cyanobacteria is globally a redox process where CO_2 is reduced to organic matter and a reducing agent is oxidized. Which is this reducing agent?

a. H_2O
b. H_2S
c. HSO_3^-
d. H_2
e. Lactate

904. Chemosynthesis, by which green sulphur bacteria fix atmospheric CO_2, is globally a redox process where CO_2 is reduced to organic matter and a reducing agent is oxidized. Which is this reducing agent?

a. H_2O
b. H_2S
c. HSO_3^-
d. H_2
e. Lactate

The chloroplast

905. Chloroplasts are particularly common in mesophyll cells close to leaf surface. Which of the following figures does most fit with the normal number of chloroplasts usually found in any of these cells?

a. 1
b. 5
c. 50
d. 500
e. 50000

906. Eukaryotic algae have chloroplasts. Which of the following figures does most fit with the normal number of chloroplasts usually found in any of these cells?

a. 1
b. 5
c. 50
d. 500
e. 50000

907. Which of the following assertions is FALSE?

a. Chloroplasts have an external membrane with a very selective permeability and an internal membrane which shows poor selectivity.
b. Chloroplasts have their own DNA, as well as ribosomes and other molecular machinery that allows them to express some of their genes.
c. The thylakoids are stacked membranous sacks located inside the chloroplast, that have chlorophyll and where photosynthesis light-dependent reactions take place.
d. The ATP and NADPH produced during light-dependent reactions are released to the stroma, where photosynthesis light-independent reactions takes place.
e. Sunlight absorption occurs in thylakoid membranes.

908. The chloroplasts of eukaryote cells very closely resemble, from an structural or functional point of view, to cyanobacteria. So much that it is very likely that they come evolutionarily from them. Which of the following bacteria species is a cyanobacteria?

a. Entamoeba hystolitica
b. Helicobacter pilory
c. Staphylococcus aureus
d. Bacillus cereus
e. Anabaena azollae

Pigments, light absorption and light-dependent reactions

909. The speed of light in vacuum is...

a. $3 \cdot 10^{-6}$ m/s
b. 3 m/s
c. $3 \cdot 10^3$ m/s
d. $3 \cdot 10^6$ m/s
e. $3 \cdot 10^8$ m/s

910. Which is the final electron acceptor in the light-dependent reactions?

a. el NADH
b. el $FADH_2$
c. el NADPH
d. el H_2O
e. el pyruvate

911. The electrons excited in photosystem II (P680 reaction center) cause an electron deficit in this system that has to be restored by an electron donor. Which is it?

a. Plastocyanin
b. Plastoquinol
c. Water
d. Light
e. Chlorophyll B

912. When the concentration of $NADP^+$ within the stroma is low, a mechanism of cyclic flux of electrons is activated, what does it consist of?

a. The electrons excited in P700 complex (photosystem I) are transferred to $NADP^+$ and from there to P680 complex (photosystem II).
b. The electrons excited in P700 complex (photosystem I) are transferred to $NADP^+$ and from there they return to P700 complex.
c. The electrons excited in P700 complex (photosystem I) are transferred to H_2O and from there they return to P700 complex.
d. The electrons excited in P700 complex (photosystem I) are transferred to plastocyanin, from there they pass to ferredoxin and from there they return to P700 complex.
e. The electrons excited in P700 complex (photosystem I) are transferred to ferredoxin and then to cytochrome b_6f, from where they return to P700 through plastocyanin.

913. The energy (E) of a photon can be obtained, if you know some parameters, by the Planck's law. How is this energy calculated according to this law? (h=Planck's constant; ν =frequency of the photon; λ=wavelength of the photon)

a. $E = (1/2) \cdot \nu^2$
b. $E = h\nu$
c. $E = h/\lambda$
d. $E = (1/2) \cdot (h/\nu)^2$
e. $E = (1/2) \cdot (\nu/h)^2$

914. The energy of a mole of photons is ocassionally measured to evaluate the amount of energy arriving to photosynthesis as a function of the wavelength of the received radiation. Approximately, which of the following values would be plausible as the value of energy per mole of photons of an ultraviolet radiation? (the letters K, M and G refer to kilo, mega and giga prefixes, respectively).

a. 3 KJ
b. 500 KJ
c. 3 MJ
d. 500 MJ
e. 3 GJ

915. The energy of a mole of photons is ocassionally measured to evaluate the amount of energy arriving to photosynthesis as a function of the wavelength of the received radiation. Approximately, what is the difference between the energy per mole of photons between two radiations located at opposite ends of visible spectrum (violet and red)?

a. 5 KJ
b. 40 KJ
c. 150 KJ
d. 400 KJ
e. 2500 KJ

916. Photosynthesis light-dependent reactions involves two photosystems, that absorb visible light mainly at two wavelengths. Which are these wavelengths?

    a. 450 and 480 nm
    b. 450 and 500 nm
    c. 540 and 600 nm
    d. 540 and 690 nm
    e. 680 and 700 nm

917. Which of the following lists is ordered from largest to smallest energy per mole of photons?

    a. blue → green → ultraviolet →yellow → infrered
    b. ultraviolet → blue → green → yellow → infrered
    c. ultraviolet → yellow → blue → green →infrered
    d. infrered → yellow → green → blue → ultraviolet
    e. infrered → green → yellow → blue → ultraviolet

918. The structure of chlorophyll is characteristic because...

    a. presents an atom of Mg^{2+} coordinated by two rings of pyridine
    b. presents an atom of Cu^{2+} coordinated by four rings of furano
    c. presents an atom of Mg^{2+} coordinated by four rings of pyrrole
    d. presents an atom of Fe^{2+} coordinated by four rings of tiofeno
    e. presents an atom of Cl^{-} coordinated by two rings of tyrosine

919. The following pigments have a maximum peak of absorption of visible light at a given wavelength between 400 and 700 nm. Which of the following lists do order the pigments from smallest to largest wavelength, when it comes to that peak?

    a. phycocyanin → chlorophyll a → β-carotene → phycoerythrin
    b. chlorophyll a → β-carotene → phycoerythrin → phycocyanin
    c. β-carotene → phycoerythrin → phycocyanin → chlorophyll a
    d. chlorophyll a → phycocyanin → β-carotene → phycoerythrin
    e. phycocyanin → β-carotene → chlorophyll a → phycoerythrin

920. Pheophytins are molecules almost identical to chlorophylls. The difference is that the central Mg^{2+} atom has been substituted in pheophytins by...

a. one Fe^{2+}
b. two Na^+
c. one Ca^{2+}
d. two Li^+
e. two protons

921. Which of the following assertions is FALSE?

a. Chlorophyll a has two absorption peaks within the visible spectrum, one at ~440 nm and another at ~680 nm.
b. Chlorophyll b has the same absorption peaks as chlorophyll a, but slightly more centered within the spectrum, one at ~490 nm and another at ~670 nm.
c. Phycocyanin absorbs with good intensity between 550 and 650 nm, having its maximum of absorption at ~620 nm.
d. Phycoerythrins have an absorption peak near 700 nm.
e. Between 500 and 600 nm, chlorophylls (both a and b) absorb very little radiation.

922. The photosystem I...

a. receives the electrons from photosystem II, after passing through several transporting molecules, and transfer them to $NADP^+$, generating NADPH.
b. generates a redox potential, necessary for the reduction of O_2 to water.
c. moves freely across thylakoid lumen.
d. produces ATP thanks to the electromotive force of the electrons passing across it.
e. transfers electrons to plastocyanin, that transport them to photosystem II, where water photodissociation takes place.

923. Visible sun radiation that arrives to Earth's surface has different intensity depending on wavelength. At which wavelength is this intensity maximum?

a. 300 nm
b. 400 nm
c. 500 nm
d. 600 nm
e. 700 nm

924. Plastocyanin is a protein that takes the electrons delivered by cytochrome b6f. It moves within thylakoid lumen and transfers them to the P700 reaction center, of photosystem I. Which redox process does occur in this protein for capture and delivery of electrons to take place?

a. The coenzyme NAD^+, non-covalently bound to plastocyanin, captures electrons, becoming $NADH+H^+$, and turns into NAD^+ when delivering them.

b. A copper atom passes from Cu^{2+} to Cu^+ when capturing an electron and converts again into Cu^{2+} when delivering it.

c. The coenzyme FAD^+, covalently bound to plastocyanin, captures electrons, becoming $FADH_2$, and turns into FAD^+ when delivering them.

d. An iron atom passes from Fe^{3+} to Fe^{2+} when capturing an electron, and turns into Fe^{3+} when delivering it.

e. Two protons of plastocyanin active site are converted into molecular hydrogen (H_2) when capturing electrons and dissociate $(2 H^+)$ when delivering them.

925. Robert Emerson and William Arnold, during 1930 decade, performed several experiments with algae of the genus *Chlorella*, arriving to an important discovery related to photosynthesis. What was it?

a. They saw that, despite this algae may act with maximum efficacy, they only produced a molecule of O_2 for each ~2500 present chlorophyll molecules, establishing the first evidences of the resonance transmission system between photosystems.

b. They observe that, in addition to chlorophyll a, other pigments like phycoerythrin or phycocyanin were present in these algae and were excited by visible light.

c. They observe that, the relation between consumed CO_2 and produced O_2 was lower than 1 (~0.8), providing the first signs that a certain amount of oxygen of CO_2 is finally converted into H_2O, as would be verified some years later by isotopic labelling.

d. They established that approximately a 40% of the absorbed sun energy was used to excite pigments different from chlorophyll (phycoerythrin and phycocyanin), which excitation did not result in net carbon fixation.

e. They observe that, if they feed algae with isotopically labelled CO_2, most of the oxygen of this gas were finally incorporated into plant glucose and not in released O_2.

926. In cyclic photophosphorylation...

a. cytochrome b_6f and ferredoxin compete by the electrons of ferredoxin.
b. cytochrome b_6f pumps H^+ into thylakoid lumen, thus enabling ATP synthesis.
c. O_2 is not released.
d. a and b are right
e. All are right

927. Hill's reactions (Robert Hill, University of Cambridge, 1939) showed that...

a. the photons received by a photosynthetic system are transmited through the chlorophyll molecules until arrive to some places named 'reaction centers'.
b. the chloroplasts, lighted up by visible light, can oxidize water to O_2 without the participation of CO_2.
c. when feeding a culture of green algae with CO_2 and iron (II) oxide (Fe^{2+}), the iron is oxidized to Fe^{3+} and the CO_2 incorporates into 5-carbon molecules.
d. when feeding a culture of green algae with CO_2 in the presence of visible light, a reactive gas called oxygen is produced.
e. when feeding a culture of green algae with CO_2 and hydrogen sulfide (H_2S), sulphur is oxidized (forming SO_2) and the CO_2 is reduced being incorporated into 6-carbon molecules (then non-identified, but that turned out to be mainly glucose).

928. Photosystem II receives the light stimulation and one of its electrons is excited. This electron is transferred to a first acceptor called...

a. pheophytin a
b. cytochrome b_6f
c. plastoquinone
d. plastocyanin
e. NADPH

929. In the cyclic photophosphorylation...

a. cytochrome b_6f and ferredoxin compete by the electrons of ferredoxin.
b. net production of NADPH and O_2 does not occur.
c. ATP synthesis is allowed, taking advantage of sunlight intensity in conditions of low concentration of oxidized precursors ($NADP^+$)
d. a and b are right
e. All are right

930. Pheophytin electrons are transferred to the...

a. photosystem I
b. cytochrome b_6f
c. plastoquinone
d. plastocyanin
e. NADPH

931. The plastoquinone reduced by the electrons coming from pheophytin a is called plastoquinol. It travels through thylakoid lipid bilayer and delivers its electrons to a protein system with several iron-sulfur clusters named...

a. cytochrome c
b. cytochrome b_6f
c. hemocyanin
d. Rieske complex
e. cytochrome f

932. Cytochrome b_6f transfers its electrons to the...

a. photosystem I
b. photosystem II
c. plastoquinone
d. plastocyanin
e. NADPH

933. Fill in the gaps:

"Electrons excited in photosystem I pass initially to a chlorophyllic acceptor (__). Afterwards they are transferred to a molecule of _____, to pass later to a set of three iron-sulfur proteins (_____, _____ and _____). Then, they arrive to soluble _____, found within the stroma, from where electrons finally arrive to _____ "

a. A_0 / phylloquinone / F_X / F_B / F_A / ferredoxin / NADPH
b. phylloquinone / A_0 / F_X / F_B / F_A / ferredoxin / NADPH
c. A_0 / ferredoxin / F_X / F_B / F_A / phylloquinone / NADPH
d. ferredoxin / NADPH / F_X / F_B / F_A / phylloquinone / A_0
e. A_0 / NADPH / F_X / F_B / F_A / ferredoxin / phylloquinone

934. The electrons transferred to the electron transport chain from photosystem I have to be restored to compensate original electron deficit. Where do these 'spare electrons' come from?

 a. From water
 b. From plastocyanin
 c. From reduced ferredoxin
 d. From CO_2
 e. From mitochondrial electron transport chain

935. All photosynthesis light-dependent reactions can be summarized in the following chemical equation, where hv stands for a photon (indicate the right option).

 a. $6\,H_2O + 6\,CO_2 + 12\,NADP^+ + 12\,H^+\ 6\,hv \rightarrow C_6H_{12}O_6 + 6\,O_2 + 12\,NADPH$
 b. $6\,H_2O + 6\,CO_2 + 6\,NADP^+ + 12\,H^+\ 6\,hv \rightarrow C_6H_{12}O_6 + 6\,O_2 + 6\,NADPH$
 c. $6\,H_2O + 6\,CO_2 + 12\,NAD^+ + 12\,H^+\ 6\,hv \rightarrow C_6H_{12}O_6 + 6\,O_2 + 12\,NADH$
 d. $2\,H_2O + 2\,NAD^+ + 4\,hv \rightarrow 2\,H^+ + O_2 + 2\,NADH$
 e. $2\,H_2O + 2\,NADP^+ + 4\,hv \rightarrow 2\,H^+ + O_2 + 2\,NADPH$

936. The joint action of photosystems I and II gives rise to...

 a. the $NADP^+$ to NADPH reduction.
 b. the acidification of thylakoid lumen in relation to stroma.
 c. the generation of a proton gradient across thylakoid membrane.
 d. a and c are right
 e. All are right

937. The gradient of protons generated in thylakoid membrane as a consequence of the functioning of photosystems I and II enables the generation of a proton flux and coupling this flux to ATP synthesis. The protein machinery that performs this process within chloroplast is similar to that dealing with the same process within mitochondria, and is named CF_0-CF_1 complex. It has been calculated how many protons have to pass across the membrane by this system to generate an ATP molecule. How many are they?

 a. 3
 b. 5
 c. 7
 d. 9
 e. 12

938. Which of the following assertions on the distribution of photosystems in the thylakoid membrane is right?

a. The thylakoid membrane that is not in direct contact with the stroma has much more photosystem I than photosystem II.
b. The thylakoid membrane that is in direct contact with the stroma has much more photosystem I than photosystem II.
c. The thylakoid membrane that is in direct contact with the stroma has much more ATP synthase complexes than the membrane that is not in direct contact with stroma.
d. b and c are right
e. All are right

939. In cyclic photophosphorylation ...

a. cytochrome b_6f and ferredoxin compete by the electrons of P680 complex.
b. NADPH is produced.
c. approximately an ATP is produced for each two electrons that complete the cycle.
d. cytochrome b_6f pumps protons from thylakoid lumen into stroma, enabling ATP synthesis.
e. O_2 is released.

Light-independent reactions. Calvin Cycle

940. Where do photosynthesis light-independent reactions take place?

a. Within the thylakoid lumen.
b. Within the thylakoid membrane.
c. Within the stroma.
d. Within the inner membrane of chloroplast.
e. Within the external membrane of chloroplast.

941. Which of the following sentences does summarize the biological role of the photosynthesis light-independent reactions?

a. To protect chlorophyll, restoring its electrons, after the intense wearing out of light-dependent reactions.
b. To fix atmospheric CO_2 in form of sugars, by using the reducing power (NADPH) and the energy (ATP) obtained in light-dependent reactions.
c. To generate ATP from the protons coming from the NADPH produced in light-dependent reactions.
d. To obtain electrons coming from H_2O to generate ATP and reducing power to be used in sugar biosynthesis.
e. To favour the extraction of water from the underground (evapotranspiration) while distributing nutrients throughout the plant.

942. Photosynthesis light-independent reactions...

a. may happen without light, but are accelerated in presence of light.
b. involve the cyclic addition of CO_2 molecules to Calvin Cycle.
c. use the chemical energy (ATP) produced in thylakoid membrane in presence of light.
d. b and c are true.
e. All are true.

943. The initial acceptor of CO_2 in Calvin cycle is ribulose-1,5-bisP. To which carbon of this molecule does initially bind CO_2?

a. 1
b. 2
c. 3
d. 4
e. 5

944. When incorporating to Calvin Cycle, the CO_2 binds to ribulose-1,5-bisP forming a 6-carbon intermediate called 2-carboxy-3-keto-D-arabinitol-1,5-bisphosphate. This intermediate is then hydrolized giving rise to two 3-carbon molecules, one of which contains the carbon just incorporated into the cycle. Which molecules are?

    a. 2 molecules of 3-phosphoglycerate
    b. 3-phosphoglycerate and 1,3-bisphosphoglycerate
    c. glyceraldehyde-3-phosphate and dihydroxyacetone phosphate
    d. pyruvate and dihydroxyacetone phosphate
    e. glyceraldehyde-3-phosphate and 1,3-bisphosphoglycerate

945. ¿Cuántas moléculas de ATP se consumen para que 1 molécula de CO_2 quede incorporada en una molécula de 3-phosphoglycerate del ciclo de Calvin?

    a. ninguna
    b. 1
    c. 2
    d. 3
    e. 4

946. In the Calvin Cycle enter 6 CO_2 for each produced glucose. For this synthesis is necessary the consumption of chemical energy (ATP) and the oxidation of NADPH. How many ATPs and NADPHs are necessary to produce a glucose?

    a. 6 ATPs and 3 NADPHs
    b. 6 ATPs and 6 NADPHs
    c. 12 ATPs and 6 NADPHs
    d. 6 ATPs and 12 NADPHs
    e. 12 ATPs and 12 NADPHs

947. The ribulose-1,5-bisphosphate oxidase (rubisco)...

    a. Is stimulated by an increase of pH.
    b. Is stimulated by an increase in [CO_2].
    c. Is inhibited by an increase in [Mg^{2+}].
    d. a and b are right.
    e. All are right.

948. When incorporating to Calvin Cycle, the CO_2 binds to ribulose-1,5-bisP forming a 6-carbon intermediate called 2-carboxy-3-keto-D-arabinitol-1,5-bisphosphate. This intermediate is then hydrolized giving rise to two 3-carbon molecules, one of which contains the carbon just incorporated into the cycle. Which enzyme does catalyse this reaction?

a. ribulose-1,5-bisP carboxylase-oxidase
b. cytochrome b_6f
c. ribulose-1,5-bisP dehydrogenase
d. ribulose-1-P carboxykinase
e. ribulose-5-P carboxykinase

949. How many molecules of NADPH are reduced to NADP$^+$ so that a CO_2 can be incorporated in a 3-phosphoglycerate molecule of Calvin Cycle?

a. None
b. 1
c. 2
d. 3
e. 4

Photorespiration and C_4 cycle

950. When is preferably activated the oxygenase activity of Rubisco?

a. in conditions of low $[O_2]$ and low $[CO_2]$
b. in conditions of high $[O_2]$ and low $[CO_2]$
c. in conditions of high [glyoxylate]
d. in conditions of low [ribulose-1,5-bisP]
e. in conditions of high [3-phosphoglycerate]

951. Photorespiration...
a. is activated when $[CO_2]$ decreases.
b. is inhibited by sunlight.
c. is inhibited when temperature rises.
d. a and c are right
e. All are right

952. The activation of photorespiration causes the production of two intermediates within the chloroplast. Which are?
a. 3-phosphoglycerate and phosphoglycolate.
b. Ribulose-1,5-bisP and hydrogen peroxide.
c. Ribulose-1,5-bisP and lactate.
d. Glycine and serine.
e. Glycine and glyoxylate.

953. The phosphoglycolate produced in some steps of photorespiration...

a. is driven to mitochondria, where it is converted into oxaloacetate and incorporates to Krebs cycle.
b. goes to cytosol, where it is transformed into phosphoenolpyruvate, that is mainly incorporated to pyruvate dehydrogenase and Krebs cycle.
c. is desphosphorylated to glycolate and reduced to glycine, that enter diverse routes of biosynthesis of amino acids.
d. is desphosphorylated to glycolate, that passes to peroxisomes and is converted into hydrogen peroxide and glyoxylate. The hydrogen peroxide is eliminated by catalase and the glyoxylate is transformed into glycine.
e. is driven to mitochondria, where, through a complex multienzymatic process, the union of two phosphoglycolates to form a serine, with the loss of CO_2 and NH_3, takes place.

954. C₄ plants...

a. perform photosynthesis without water photodissociation.
b. incorporate the 4-carbon intermediates of Calvin Cycle to Krebs cycle mainly as oxaloacetate.
c. have an additional photosynthetic route that allow a more efficient use of the CO_2 produced in photorespiration.
d. do not perform photorespiration.
e. incorporate the CO_2 to short-chain amino acids to produce complex amino acids.

955. Which of the following assertions is FALSE?

a. C₄ plants reduce the losses due to photorespiration by a pathway complementary to Calvin Cycle.
b. Phosphoenolpyruvate carboxylase, in C₄ plants, has an affinity for CO_2 higher than rubisco.
c. In C₄ plants, the most internal cells perform the Calvin Cycle with the CO_2 provided by mesophyll cells mesófilas, closer to leaf surface.
d. In C₄ plants, in mesophyll cells, CO_2 is added to phosphoenolpyruvate, forming oxaloacetate that, then, is converted into malate, passing to most internal cells.
e. Phosphoenolpyruvate carboxylase of C₄ plants, as well as rubisco, has an oxygenase activity that is activated at low CO_2 concentrations.

956. This diagram represents the cycle of C₄ plants. What do A, B, C and D letters stand for?

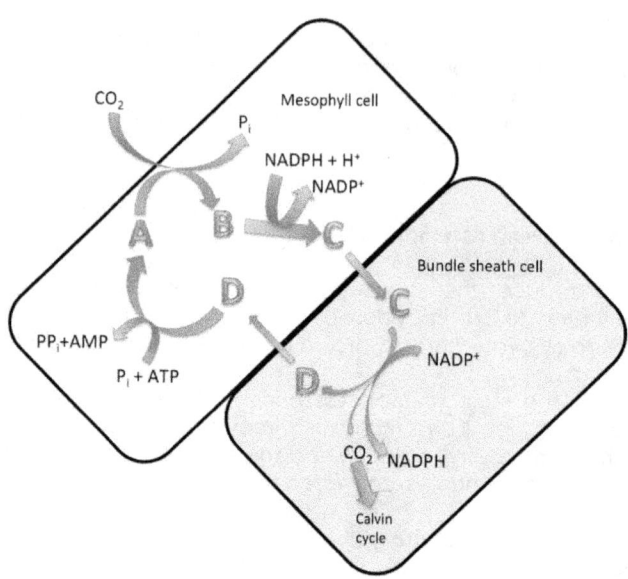

a. A=pyruvate; B=phosphoenolpyruvate; C=lactate; D=citrate
b. A=ribulose-1,5-bisP; B=3-phosphoglycerate; C=pyruvate; D=malate
c. A=phosphoenolpyruvate; B=oxaloacetate; C=malate; D=pyruvate
d. A=malate; B=pyruvate; C=phosphoenolpyruvate; D=oxaloacetate
e. A=dihydroxyacetone phosphate; B=pyruvate; C=acetylCoA; D=ATP

Usual general biochemistry practices

957. The Beer-Lambert law relates the absorbance of a solution with the concentration of a given substance. It is expressed as follows...

$$\log I0/I = \varepsilon \cdot c \cdot l$$

where I_0 is the intensity of the ____ light, I is the intensity of the ___ light, ε is the ____, c the _____ of the substance and l the _____ of the sample.

 a. incident / transmitted / path length / absorption coefficient / concentration
 b. incident / transmitted / absorption coefficient / concentration / path length
 c. transmitted / incident / path length / absorption coefficient / concentration
 d. transmitted / incident / absorption coefficient / concentration / path length
 e. transmitted / incident / concentration / absorption coefficient / path length

958. Which of the following assertions, on spectrophotometry, is FALSE?

 a. The absorbance is a measure of the quantity of light that passes through the solution.
 b. The Beer-Lambert law can only be applied if we consider that the particles of the solute are randomly oriented.
 c. The Beer-Lambert law can only be applied if we consider that the incident light is monochromatic.
 d. The molar extinction coefficient varies with the nature of the solute.
 e. The molar extinction coefficient varies with the nature of the solvent.

959. Normally, in a biochemistry laboratory, the conservation solution, where the electrode of the pH meter has to be immersed at rest, has a pH of...

 a. 1
 b. 3
 c. 5
 d. 7
 e. 9

960. Which of the following assertions is FALSE?

a. When progressively adding salt (i.e. ammonium sulfate) to a protein solution, the solubility of proteins increases until achieving a maximum value, if more salt is added from this point, the proteins begin to precipitate.

b. Blue Coomassie dye (the main active agent in Bradford's reactive) colours protein solutions binding preferably to thei basic amino acids (in particular, arginine) and aromatic.

c. In an electrophoresis, positively charged particles move towards the anode and negatively charged ones move towards the cathode.

d. In an electrophoresis, the larger particles will move slower than the smaller ones, provided that the sign and magnitude of electrical charge is the same for both.

e. In the making of a polyacrylamide gel, acrylamide and bis-acrylamide polymerization is enhanced by ammonium persulfate and stabilized by the TEMED (tetramethylethylenediamine).

961. The SDS...

a. is a detergent used in protein separation by polyacrylamide gels.

b. is negatively charged.

c. binds proteins in a way almost proportional to their mass. Approximately, under saturation conditions, 1.4 g of SDS binds 1 g of protein.

d. b and c are right

e. All are right

962. When applying an electrical current to a solution, the solute molecules charged _____ migrate towards the _____, and the ones charged _____ migrate towards the ___.

a. negatively, cathode, positively, anode

b. negatively, anode, positively, cathode

c. with a net charge, cathode, negatively, anode

d. neutrally, cathode, positively, anode

e. neutrally, anode, negativelly, cathode

963. The electrophoretic mobility (μ) of a particle...

a. the quotient between the charge of the particle and its coefficient of friction

b. the quocient between the charge of the particle and the electric field

c. the quocient between the velocity of the particle and the electric field

d. the product between the charge and the speed of the particle

e. b and c are right

964. The unit of measure for the sedimentation coefficient is...

a. Newton / s^2
b. Svedberg
c. Watts / s
d. Siemens
e. m / s

965. Every particle, when following a circular trajectory supports a centrifugal force. The magnitude of this force...

a. increases as the distance to the center of the circumference also increases.
b. increases as the angular velocity of the movement decreases.
c. increases as the density of the solution where it is immersed also increases.
d. increases as the specific volume of the particle also increases.
e. a and d are right

966. The factor of flotation is...

a. the inverse of the product between the specific volume of the particle and the density of the solution
b. the difference between the specific volume of the particle and the density of the solution
c. the quotient between the specific volume of the particle and the density of the solution
d. the quotient between the density of the solution and the specific volume of the particle
e. the difference between 1 and the product between the specific volume of the particle and the density of the solution

967. In a centrifugation process...

a. if the density of a particle equals the density of the solution, the centrifugal force on the particle and so its sedimentation rate will be maximum.
b. if the density of a particle equals the density of the solution, the centrifugal force on the particle will be null and so it will not sediment.
c. if the density of a particle equals the density of the solution, the factor of flotation of the particle will be zero.
d. b and c are right
e. a and c are right

968. The factor of flotation is...

a. the product between the density of the particle and the density of the solution.
b. the quotient between the density of the particle and the density of the solution.
c. 1 minus the quotient between the density of the particle and the density of the solution.
d. 1 minus the quotient between the density of the solution and the density of the particle.
e. 1 minus the product between the density of the solution and the density of the particle.

969. The sedimentation coefficient of a particle is...
a. the quotient between the velocity of the particle and the intensity of the centrifugal field, that is the product of the radius and the square angular velocity.
b. the quotient between the coefficient of friction and the product of tha factor of flotation and the mass of the particle.
c. the inverse of the quotient indicated in the option b.
d. a and b are right
e. a and c are right

970. The unit to measure sedimentation coefficient is the Svedberg (S). 1 S equals...

a. 10^{-10} s
b. 10^{-11} s
c. 10^{-12} s
d. 10^{-13} s
e. 10^{-14} s

971. We perform an ion exchange chromatography, using an anionic resin as the stationary phase. As mobile phase we use a saline solution with crescent concentrations of sodium ([Na$^+$] is low for the initial fractions and progressively increases when we arrive to the final fractions).

After collecting the fractions of the mobile phase, we obtain the concentrations for A, B and C molecules as represented in the following diagram.

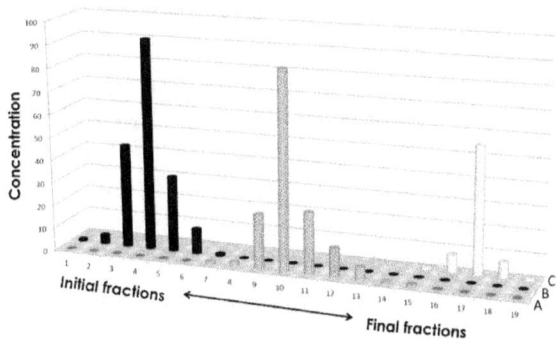

If we know that one of the molecules is negatively charged, another has a weak positive charge, and the other has a very strong positive charge, which is each molecule?

a. A=negative; B=weakly positive; C=positive
b. A=positive; B= weakly positive; C=negative
c. A= weakly positive; B=negative; C=positive
d. A= weakly positive; B=positive; C=negative
e. A=positive; B=negative; C= weakly positive

972. Proteins have an absorbance maximum at a wavelength of 270-290 nm. This is due to the absorption produced by...

a. the lateral chains of phenylalanine, tyrosine and tryptophan
b. the lateral chains of glutamic acid and aspartic acid
c. the lateral chains of valine, isoleucine, leucine and alanine
d. the lateral chains of lysine and arginine
e. the bonds of the main peptide chain

973. Proteins have an absorbance maximum at a wavelength of 180-220 nm. This is due to the absorption produced by...

a. the lateral chains of phenylalanine, tyrosine and tryptophan
b. the lateral chains of glutamic acid and aspartic acid
c. the lateral chains of valine, isoleucine, leucine and alanine
d. the lateral chains of lysine and arginine
e. the bonds of the main peptide chain

974. The extinction coefficient for a given protein at a wavelength of 200 nm...

a. ...varies as a function of protein conformation
b. ...varies as a function of the number of amino acids of the protein
c. ...varía as a function of the nature of the amino acids composing the protein
d. a, b and c are right
e. b and c are right, a is false

975. This diagram shows the functioning of a normal spectrophotometer.

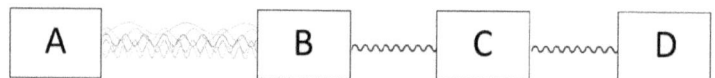

The letters A, B, C and D correspond to...

a. A = light source; B = detector; C = cuvette with the sample; D = monochromator
b. A = cuvette with the sample; B = detector; C = monochromator; D = light source
c. A = monochromator; B = light source; C = cuvette with the sample; D = detector
d. A = light source; B = cuvette with the sample; C = monochromator; D = detector
e. A = light source; B = monochromator; C = cuvette with the sample; D = detector

976. The function of the monochromator is to...

a. achieve that the incident radiation may have a constant intensity
b. achieve that the incident radiation may have an intensity higher than light source
c. achieve that the incident radiation may have an intensity lower than light source
d. maintain the intensity of incident radiation very close to light source
e. prevent the radiation with a wavelength lower than 200 nm to reach the sample

977. This diagram shows the functioning of an spectrophotometer.

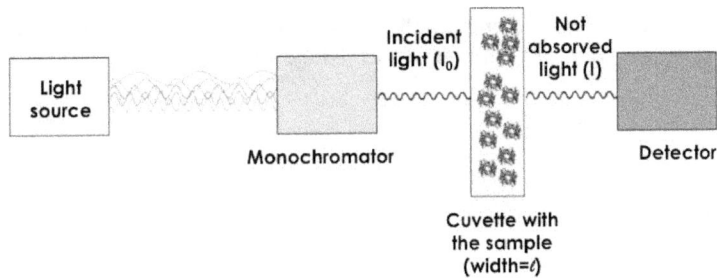

The intensity of incident radiation is I_0, the intensity of the radiation non-absorbed by the sample I, the wavelength of the incident radiation is λ. So, the absorbance (A) for a given λ is expressed by the following equation...

a. $A = \log (I_0/I)$
b. $A = \ln (I_0/I)$
c. $A = \log (I/I_0)$
d. $A = \ln (I/I_0)$
e. $A = \log (I_0 - I)$

978. NADH absorbs with quite intensity at a certain wavelength, at which NAD+ absorbs very little. This offers the possibility of using this wavelength to measure the progress of redox reactions where this pair of coenzymes participate. Which is this wavelength?

a. 340 nm
b. 380 nm
c. 420 nm
d. 460 nm
e. 500 nm

979. The absorbance can be related with the concentration (C) of a given protein by the Beer-Lambert law. If we consider I_0 and I as the incident and outgoing intensities, respectively, and ε is the molar extinction coefficient for a given wavelength, this law relates absorbance and concentration by the following equation:

a. $A = \varepsilon \cdot C$
b. $A = (I_0/I) \cdot \varepsilon \cdot C$
c. $A = \log (I_0/I) \cdot (\varepsilon / C)$
d. $A = (I_0 \cdot \varepsilon) - (I \cdot C)$
e. $A = \varepsilon / C$

980. Which of the following assertions is FALSE?

a. Hydrogen has an stable isotope ($^2H_1$ or deuterium) and a radioactive isotope ($^3H_1$ or tritium).
b. The incorporation of an stable isotope to a compound generally entails an increase of its molecular weight.
c. The ^{15}N is an stable (non-radioactive) isotope of nitrogen.
d. ^{131}I is a radioactive isotope of iodine that produces γ radiation.
e. A β ray is a high energy photon.

981. The unit of radioactive disintegration is...

a. the curie (Ci)
b. the bequerel (Bq)
c. the watt (W)
d. the einstenium (En)
e. the joule $\cdot$ mole^{-1}

982. Given a sample with a radioactivity of 0.6 μCi, how many counts per minute would be measured by an apparatus with a 25% efficiency? (1 Ci $= 2.22 \cdot 10^{12}$ desintegrations per minute)

a. 1.33 cpm
b. $1.33 \cdot 10^6$ cpm
c. $0.33 \cdot 10^{12}$ cpm
d. $0.33 \cdot 10^6$ cpm
e. $0.66 \cdot 10^{12}$ cpm

983. Which of the following expressions does correspond to the radioactive disintegration law and, so, enables to calculate the amount of a given isotope that will remain after a disintegration time? N_0 is the number of radioactive atoms of a given isotope at a time 0, t is the time and γ Is the radioactive disintegration constant for this particular isotope.

A $N = N_0 t e^{\gamma/2}$

B $N = N_0 e^{-\gamma t}$

C $N = N_0 (e^{\gamma/2t})/2$

D $N = N_0 t e^{-\gamma}$

E $N = N_0 + N_0 t + ((e^{\gamma/2t})/2)$

a. A
b. B
c. C
d. D
e. E

984. A curie is defined as...

a. the quantity of radioactivity equivalent to the one existing in 1 kg of radium.
b. the quantity of radioactivity equivalent to the one existing in 1 g of radium.
c. the quantity of radioactivity equivalent to the one existing in 1 kg of uranium.
d. the quantity of radioactivity equivalent to 1000 disintegrations per minute.
e. the quantity of radioactivity equivalent to 1 disintegration per minute.

History of biochemistry

985. In the olden days, water was considered as a chemical element. It was in 1781 when it was discovered that it was a composed substance and not a single element. Who was the author of this discovery?

a. Antoine-Laurent de Lavoisier
b. James Watt
c. Isaac Newton
d. Claude Bernard
e. Henry Cavendish

986. Which of the following assertions on myoglobin is right?

a. It was firstly described in the middle of 20th century
b. It was firstly purified in 1958, by John Kendrew
c. Its 3D structure was solved by X-ray in 1958, by Max Perutz
d. The discovery of its 3D structure deserved the Nobel Prize in Chemistry in 1962
e. Its 3D structure was described only 1 year after the one of hemoglobin

987. The model of DNA tridimensional structure, as a dextrorotary double helix, was firstly proposed by...

a. Lavoisier in the 19th century.
b. Watson and Crick in 1953.
c. Stanley Miller in 1953.
d. Jacob Schleiden in 1918.
e. Santiago Ramón y Cajal in 1906.

988. Robert Emerson and William Arnold, during 1930 decade, performed several experiments with algae of the genus *Chlorella*, arriving to an important discovery related to photosynthesis. What was it?

a. They saw that, despite this algae may act with maximum efficacy, they only produced a molecule of O_2 for each ~2500 present chlorophyll molecules, establishing the first evidences of the resonance transmission system between photosystems.

b. They observe that, in addition to chlorophyll a, other pigments like phycoerythrin or phycocyanin were present in these algae and were excited by visible light.

c. They observe that, the relation between consumed CO_2 and produced O_2 was lower than 1 (~0.8), providing the first signs that a certain amount of oxygen of CO_2 is finally converted into H_2O, as would be verified some years later by isotopic labelling.

d. They established that approximately a 40% of the absorbed sun energy was used to excite pigments different from chlorophyll (phycoerythrin and phycocyanin), which excitation did not result in net carbon fixation.

e. They observe that, if they feed algae with isotopically labelled CO_2, most of the oxygen of this gas were finally incorporated into plant glucose and not in released O_2.

989. Rosalynd Franklin...

a. performed the first assays by electrophoresis that allowed to know the protein composition of human blood.

b. collaborated with Stanley Miller and Joan Oró in the determination of the necessary conditions so as to generate organic matter from inorganic through thermoelectrical discharges.

c. developed the PCR technique for the amplification of DNA sequences by the action of Taq polymerase.

d. stood out by her studies on the allosteric modulation of hemoglobin by 2,3-bisphosphoglycerate.

e. obtained the named 'photograph 51', an image of X-ray diffraction on DNA crystals, that was essential for Watson and Crick to propose in 1953 their hypothesis on DNA tridimensional structure.

990. In 1804, two scientists showed that water was composed by two volumes of hydrogen and one of oxygen. Who were them?
a. Antoine-Laurent de Lavoisier and Henry Cavendish
b. Joseph Louis Gauy-Lussac and Alexander von Humboldt
c. Isaac Newton and Robert Hooke
d. Henry Moseley and Dmtri Mendeleiev
e. Stephen Boltzmman and Jaques Dobbereiner

991. The knowledge about neuron excitability, by action potentials, nervous impulse transmission, etc. began to be developed thanks to some very elaborated initial studies that use _____ as material, where they introduced electrodes to register excitabilities, etc.

    a. neuron axons of swordfish
    b. neuron axons of *Drosophila*
    c. neuron axons of flatworms
    d. neuron axons of least weasel
    e. neuron axons of squid

992. Fluid mosaic model, on biological membranes, was proposed in 1972 by...

    a. S.J. Singer and G.L. Nicholson
    b. S. Miller and J. Oró
    c. P. Mitchell
    d. J. Watson and F. Crick
    e. F. Burlington and M. Perutz

993. Louis Pasteur observed a behaviour in the glycolytic pathway known today as 'Pasteur effect' What is it about?

    a. Glycolysis stopped in presence of strong acids
    b. While yeasts are degrading glucose, they are exposed to crescent concentrations of ethanol, thus deriving glycolytic pathway towards lactate production
    c. The rate of glycolytic pathway is higher in yeasts that are simultaneously feeded with fatty acids
    d. Adding ethanol to a yeast cell culture results in an accumulation of pyruvate and stops glycolytic pathway
    e. The rate of glycolysis drastically drops when the culture of yeasts is exposed to air

994. Fritz Lipmann received, together with Hans Krebs, the Nobel prize in the first half of the 20th century. Krebs was awarded for discovering that some organic compounds degradate in a cyclic route. What was the most known discovery made by Fritz Lipmann?

    a. coenzyme A
    b. tricarboxylic acids cycle
    c. citric acid cycle
    d. b and c
    e. the anaerobic degradation of pyruvate into lactate

995. In the experiments of Hans Krebs with muscular tissue of pigeon, what effects were observed after adding citrate to this tissue?

a. an increase in pyruvate oxidation proportional to the amount of added citrate
b. a reduction in O_2 consumption proportional to the amount of added citrate
c. a decrease in pyruvate oxidation proportional to the amount of added citrate
d. an increase in O_2 consumption proportional to the amount of added citrate
e. an increase in O_2 consumption extremely high if compared to the amount of added citrate

996. In the study of vitamins, are known the works of a Polish biochemist called Casimir Funk. Which of the following is one of his contributions?

a. He observed that some diseases like beriberi, pellagra, scurvy or rickets were caused by a food deficiency of a substance that he named vitamin ('the amine of life'), bringing this to the term 'vitamin' for these substances.
b. He discovered the role of folic acid in the prevention of neural tube defects.
c. He indicated that the accumulation of tricarboxylic acids within cells that performed glycolysis in aerobic conditions was much higher in the presence of thiamine pyrophosphate (TPP), thus originally establishing the role of this coenzyme in sugar metabolism.
d. He described the importance of retinoic acid in the processes of cell regeneration.
e. He discovered that the enzyme L-gulonolactone oxidase (essential for vitamin C synthesis), present in many animals, was not functional in humans. This explained why this vitamin has an essential character for people, whereas it is not needed in the diet of other mamals, a fact that was anciently known.

997. Hill's reactions (Robert Hill, University of Cambridge, 1939) showed that...

a. the photons received by a photosynthetic system are transmited through the chlorophyll molecules until arrive to some places named *'reaction centers'*.
b. the chloroplasts, lighted up by visible light, can oxidize water to O_2 without the participation of CO_2.
c. when feeding a culture of green algae with CO_2 and iron (II) oxide (Fe^{2+}), the iron is oxidized to Fe^{3+} and the CO_2 incorporates into 5-carbon molecules.
d. when feeding a culture of green algae with CO_2 in the presence of visible light, a reactive gas called oxygen is produced.
e. when feeding a culture of green algae with CO_2 and hydrogen sulfide (H_2S), sulphur is oxidized (forming SO_2) and the CO_2 is reduced being incorporated into 6-carbon molecules (then non-identified, but that turned out to be mainly glucose).

998. At the beginning of 20th century (1904) a series of very complete experiments performed by a German chemist, by using the methyl → phenyl substitution as metabolic tracer and overtaking to the appearing of radioactive tracers, allow to dilucidate the pathway of fatty acids within eukaryotic cells. Who was this chemist?

    a. Lothar Andgewante
    b. Franz Knoop
    c. Feodor Lynen
    d. Adouls Diels-Alder
    e. Frederick Wittig

999. Von Mering and Minkowski were two physicians of the second half of 19th century to whom an important discovery on metabolism is attributed. Which is it?

    a. They demonstrated that the pancreas disfunction was related to diabetes generation.
    b. They isolated the ATP as intermediate in most of the chemical energy transactions within the body.
    c. They demonstrated that the heme group was degraded in the liver generating bilirubin.
    d. They proof that phosphofructokinase-I was an important check-point for the control of the flux of glycolysis.
    e. They described that ribose-5-P, coming from pentose phosphate pathway, was the main precursor in the endogenous purine biosynthesis.

1000. In 1806, the French chemists Louis-Nicolas Vauquelin and Pierre Jean Robiquet, isolated from a plant the first known amino acid. Which is it?

    a. asparagine
    b. glycine
    c. alanine
    d. phenylalanine
    e. threonine

References

The presented multiple-choice question collection arises from an exhaustive and deep review of the following reference books of General and Medical Biochemistry.

Baynes, J. W. and Dominiczak M. H. (2009) "Medical Biochemistry" 3rd edition (Mosby, St. Louis)

Berg, J. M. et al. (2010) "Biochemistry" 7th edition (W.H. Freeman, New York)

Devlin, T. M. (2010). "Textbook of biochemistry with clinical correlations" 7th edition (John Wiley & Sons, West Sussex)

Feduchi Canosa, E. and otros (2010) "Bioquímica: conceptos esenciales" 1st edition (Editorial Médica Panamericana, Madrid)

Ferrier, D.R. (2013) "Biochemistry" 6th edition (Lippincott Williams and Wilkins, Hagerstown)

Hicks, J.J. (2007) "Bioquímica" 2nd edition (Editorial Interamericana McGraw-Hill, México)

Koolman, J. and Rohn, KH (2012) "Bioquímica humana: texto and atlas" 4th edition (Editorial Médica Panamericana, Madrid)

Manzoul, S. M. (2010) "Biochemistry" 2nd edition (McGraw-Hill, UK)

McKee, T. and McKee J. R. (2009) "Biochemistry" 4th edition (Editorial Interamericana McGraw-Hill, México)

Mathews, C.K. et al. (2012) "Bioquímica" 4th edition (Pearson, Toronto)

Murray, R.K. et al. (2012) "Harper's illustrated biochemistry" 29th edition (McGraw-Hill, UK)

Nelson, D.L. and Cox, M.M. (2012) "Lehninger Principles of Biochemistry" 6th edition (W.H. Freeman, New York)

Voet, D., Voet, J. G. and Pratt, C. W. (2012) "Principles of Biochemistry" 4th edition (John Wiley & Sons, West Sussex)

Answers

1d	43e	85a	127b	169d	211b	253e
2c	44d	86e	128d	170b	212c	254e
3d	45c	87e	129b	171a	213d	255b
4e	46a	88b	130e	172a	214a	256e
5d	47a	89a	131e	173a	215e	257d
6c	48c	90d	132a	174a	216a	258d
7a	49b	91b	133d	175b	217d	259b
8b	50a	92e	134e	176e	218c	260a
9c	51d	93d	135b	177d	219e	261e
10b	52e	94e	136d	178d	220e	262c
11b	53c	95b	137b	179b	221e	263a
12a	54e	96c	138e	180a	222b	264a
13a	55b	97d	139d	181a	223a	265b
14c	56d	98c	140c	182b	224c	266e
15a	57e	99c	141c	183d	225e	267d
16e	58d	100a	142d	184c	226c	268a
17e	59a	101d	143d	185b	227e	269b
18b	60e	102c	144c	186c	228a	270a
19b	61d	103e	145e	187e	229a	271c
20d	62b	104a	146e	188d	230a	272d
21d	63b	105c	147b	189a	231c	273b
22a	64d	106c	148d	190c	232d	274b
23e	65d	107a	149b	191a	233c	275b
24a	66b	108a	150d	192d	234d	276a
25e	67d	109c	151a	193e	235b	277e
26a	68a	110b	152d	194b	236c	278c
27c	69b	111a	153e	195a	237e	279d
28b	70e	112b	154d	196d	238e	280c
29a	71e	113b	155b	197a	239c	281a
30a	72d	114e	156d	198a	240d	282b
31b	73e	115c	157b	199d	241e	283e
32b	74a	116a	158d	200e	242a	284d
33e	75b	117d	159a	201d	243b	285d
34d	76c	118e	160d	202d	244e	286a
35e	77d	119b	161d	203a	245e	287d
36a	78a	120b	162b	204e	246d	288d
37c	79e	121d	163a	205c	247a	289b
38b	80c	122a	164e	206b	248d	290d
39d	81e	123e	165e	207a	249a	291e
40e	82c	124b	166a	208a	250e	292e
41a	83b	125c	167c	209c	251d	293d
42d	84c	126b	168c	210e	252c	294a

295c	341b	387e	433e	479a	525d	571c
296d	342d	388a	434a	480d	526d	572b
297e	343a	389a	435b	481d	527e	573b
298b	344b	390e	436c	482d	528c	574b
299a	345b	391d	437c	483e	529c	575c
300b	346a	392a	438c	484a	530e	576e
301d	347b	393b	439d	485a	531b	577e
302b	348d	394d	440b	486b	532e	578d
303a	349a	395b	441c	487e	533b	579d
304e	350e	396d	442e	488c	534e	580c
305a	351c	397b	443b	489c	535e	581a
306a	352e	398a	444a	490c	536b	582e
307d	353b	399d	445c	491c	537d	583c
308b	354a	400e	446b	492d	538d	584b
309d	355d	401c	447a	493a	539a	585a
310e	356a	402d	448e	494a	540d	586c
311d	357c	403d	449b	495d	541b	587d
312a	358b	404b	450e	496e	542c	588b
313d	359a	405e	451b	497a	543a	589e
314d	360a	406d	452e	498b	544c	590a
315b	361b	407b	453e	499b	545b	591b
316e	362b	408a	454d	500c	546b	592a
317b	363b	409d	455a	501b	547e	593d
318b	364c	410a	456a	502e	548d	594e
319b	365a	411a	457a	503e	549d	595a
320b	366b	412d	458a	504e	550a	596d
321d	367b	413e	459c	505b	551e	597d
322a	368e	414c	460a	506d	552b	598a
323a	369a	415e	461b	507a	553a	599e
324e	370d	416d	462a	508b	554c	600e
325b	371c	417c	463d	509a	555e	601c
326c	372d	418a	464e	510a	556b	602b
327a	373d	419b	465a	511e	557b	603a
328b	374b	420c	466a	512a	558c	604a
329b	375a	421d	467d	513c	559b	605d
330c	376c	422a	468e	514e	560a	606a
331e	377c	423d	469c	515b	561c	607a
332c	378b	424a	470e	516e	562b	608e
333c	379a	425c	471d	517b	563c	609c
334a	380c	426b	472c	518c	564a	610a
335b	381b	427e	473e	519b	565a	611a
336d	382c	428b	474a	520b	566d	612e
337d	383c	429e	475e	521b	567b	613b
338d	384c	430a	476b	522e	568a	614e
339e	385d	431d	477d	523a	569a	615b
340e	386b	432e	478e	524e	570b	616b

617a	663b	709b	755d	801a	847b	893b
618e	664b	710a	756c	802a	848a	894d
619b	665a	711b	757c	803d	849c	895e
620e	666c	712d	758a	804c	850b	896e
621e	667a	713e	759a	805a	851c	897e
622e	668a	714d	760b	806c	852b	898c
623b	669b	715a	761d	807a	853a	899c
624a	670d	716e	762a	808e	854a	900b
625d	671c	717c	763b	809b	855b	901a
626b	672a	718e	764b	810e	856e	902c
627a	673e	719b	765c	811d	857b	903a
628d	674a	720b	766b	812e	858a	904b
629b	675b	721e	767d	813e	859e	905c
630a	676c	722b	768d	814b	860a	906a
631c	677c	723b	769d	815e	861e	907a
632d	678d	724d	770b	816a	862e	908e
633a	679e	725c	771e	817c	863a	909e
634b	680d	726b	772b	818d	864b	910c
635d	681d	727b	773b	819e	865d	911c
636d	682b	728c	774b	820b	866e	912e
637a	683b	729e	775a	821a	867e	913b
638a	684b	730e	776d	822a	868c	914b
639e	685d	731a	777e	823c	869e	915c
640c	686d	732b	778c	824e	870a	916e
641c	687a	733b	779b	825a	871d	917b
642b	688a	734b	780b	826a	872a	918c
643a	689b	735a	781b	827e	873d	919b
644e	690c	736e	782a	828d	874a	920e
645c	691e	737e	783b	829e	875c	921d
646d	692b	738c	784c	830e	876e	922a
647b	693a	739a	785a	831c	877e	923c
648e	694c	740a	786a	832e	878c	924b
649e	695a	741e	787d	833d	879b	925a
650d	696c	742c	788e	834d	880e	926e
651b	697d	743b	789c	835a	881e	927b
652a	698d	744a	790e	836c	882a	928a
653b	699c	745e	791e	837b	883a	929e
654c	700b	746a	792b	838e	884a	930c
655a	701c	747a	793d	839a	885e	931b
656d	702d	748d	794a	840d	886a	932d
657e	703d	749a	795d	841e	887b	933a
658a	704c	750a	796a	842c	888c	934b
659a	705c	751e	797a	843a	889d	935e
660d	706a	752b	798a	844e	890b	936e
661e	707b	753d	799c	845d	891a	937a
662e	708d	754e	800a	846d	892e	938d

939c	948a	957b	966e	975e	984b	993e
940c	949c	958a	967d	976d	985e	994a
941b	950b	959b	968d	977a	986d	995e
942e	951a	960c	969d	978a	987b	996a
943b	952a	961e	970d	979e	988a	997b
944a	953d	962b	971c	980e	989e	998b
945c	954c	963e	972a	981a	990b	999a
946e	955e	964b	973e	982d	991e	1000a
947d	956c	965a	974d	983b	992a	

www.ingramcontent.com/pod-product-compliance
Lightning Source LLC
Chambersburg PA
CBHW051625170526
45167CB00001B/58